Get ahead!

surgery

250 SBAs for Finals

Second edition

Get ahead!

surgery
250 SBAs for Finals
Second edition

Victoria Pegna MB BS, MSc, MRCS,
Bristol Royal Infirmary, Bristol
Dominic Teichmann MB BS, BSc, MRCS,
Urology Specialist Registrar,
University Hospital of Wales, Cardiff
Theepa Nicholls MRCGP,
General Practitioner, Morecambe Surgery,
Edmonton, London
Saran Shantikumar MRCS, BHF,
Clinical Fellow, Bristol Heart Institute, Bristol

Series Editor:
Saran Shantikumar

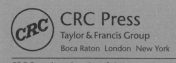

CRC Press
Taylor & Francis Group
Boca Raton London New York

CRC Press is an imprint of the
Taylor & Francis Group, an **informa** business

CRC Press
Taylor & Francis Group
6000 Broken Sound Parkway NW, Suite 300
Boca Raton, FL 33487-2742

© 2015 by Victoria Pegna, Dominic Teichmann, Theepa Nicholls, Saran Shantikumar
CRC Press is an imprint of Taylor & Francis Group, an Informa business

No claim to original U.S. Government works

Printed on acid-free paper
Version Date: 20140826

International Standard Book Number-13: 978-1-4822-5732-8 (Paperback)

Library of Congress Cataloging-in-Publication Data

Pegna, Victoria , author.
  Get ahead! Surgery : 250 SBAs for finals / authors, Victoria Pegna, Dominic Teichmann, Theepa Nicholls, Saran Shantikumar. -- Second edition.
    p. ; cm. -- (Get ahead!)
  Includes bibliographical references and index.
  ISBN 978-1-4822-5732-8 (pbk. : alk. paper) I. Teichmann, Dominic, author. II. Nicholls, Theepa, author. III. Shantikumar, Saran, author. IV. Title. V. Title: Surgery, 250 SBAs for finals. VI. Series: Get ahead! (CRC Press)
  [DNLM: 1. Surgical Procedures, Operative--Examination Questions. WO 18.2]

  RD37.2
  617.0076--dc23   2014027805

Visit the Taylor & Francis Web site at
http://www.taylorandfrancis.com

and the CRC Press Web site at
http://www.crcpress.com

Contents

Preface

Welcome to *Get ahead! SURGERY*. This book contains 250 Single Best Answer (SBA) questions covering various topics within clinical surgery. These are arranged as five practice papers, each containing 50 questions. Allow yourself 60 to 90 minutes for each paper. You can either work through the practice papers systematically or dip in and out of the book using the index as a guide to where questions on a specific topic can be found. We have tried to include all the main conditions about which you can be expected to know, as well as some more detailed knowledge suitable for candidates aiming towards distinction. As in the real exam, these papers have no preset pass mark. Whether you pass or fail depends on the distribution of scores across the whole year group, but around 60% should be sufficient.

We hope this book fulfils its aim in being a useful, informative revision aid. If you have any feedback or suggestions, please let us know (RevisionForMedicalFinals@gmail.com).

We would also like to acknowledge the help of Stephen Clausard, Development Editor at CRC Press, for his patience and proactivity in commissioning and supporting this edition and others in the *Get Ahead!* series.

Victoria Pegna
Dominic Teichmann
Theepa Nicholls
Saran Shantikumar

Introduction to *Get ahead!*

GET AHEAD!

Single Best Answer questions (SBAs) are becoming more popular as a method of assessment in summative medical school examinations. Each clinical vignette is followed by a list of five possible answers, of which only one is correct. SBAs have the advantage of testing candidates' knowledge of clinical scenarios rather than their ability at detailed factual recall. However, they do not always parallel real-life situations and are no comparison to clinical decision-making. Either way, the SBA is here to stay.

The *Get ahead!* series is aimed primarily at undergraduate finalists. Much like the real exam, we have endeavoured to include commonly asked questions as well as a generous proportion of harder stems, appropriate for the more ambitious student aiming for honours. The Medical Schools Council Assessment Alliance (MSCAA) is a partnership aiming to improve assessment practice between all undergraduate medical schools in the UK. The questions in the *Get ahead!* series are written to follow the style of the MSCAA SBAs, and hence are of a similar format to what many of you can expect in your exams. All the questions in the *Get ahead!* series are accompanied by explanatory answers, including a succinct summary of the key features of each condition. Even when you get an answer right, I strongly suggest you read these – I guarantee that you'll learn something. For added interest we have included details of eponymous conditions ('eponymous' from Greek *epi* = upon + *onyma* = name; 'giving name') and, as you have just seen, some derivations of words from the original Latin or Greek.

HOW TO PASS YOUR EXAMS

The clinical scenarios given in SBAs are intended to be based on 'house officer knowledge'. Sadly this is not always the case and you shouldn't be surprised when you get a question concerning the underlying histology of testicular tumours (as I was). So start revising early and don't restrict yourself to the given syllabus if you can avoid it. If your exam is only two weeks away then CRAM, CRAM, CRAM – you'll be surprised at how much you can learn in a fortnight.

During the exam...

1. Try to answer the questions without looking at the responses first – the questions are written such that this should be possible.
2. Take your time to read the questions fully. There are no bonus marks available for finishing the paper early.
3. If you get stuck on a question then make sure that you mark down your best guess before you move on. You may not have time to return to it at the end.
4. Answer all the questions – there is no negative marking. If you are unsure, go with your instinct – it's probably going to be your best guess.
5. Never think that the examiner is trying to catch you out. Red herrings are not allowed, so don't assume there is one. If a question looks easy, it probably is!

But all this is obvious and there is no substitute for learning the material thoroughly and practicing as many questions as you can. With this book, you're off to a good start!

A final word...

The *Get ahead!* series is written by junior doctors who have recently finished finals and who have experience teaching students. As such, I hope that the books cover information that is valuable and relevant to you as undergraduates who are about to sit finals.

   I wish you the best of luck in your exams!

Saran Shantikumar
Series Editor, Get ahead!

Practice Paper 1: Questions

1. ARTERIAL BLOOD GASES (1)

A 60-year-old man develops shortness of breath and a cough productive of purulent sputum three days after a right hemicolectomy. An arterial blood gas shows pH 7.42, pO_2 7.1, pCO_2 5.2, bicarbonate 25.

Reference ranges: pO_2 >11.0 kPa, pCO_2 4.6–6.0 kPa, bicarbonate 22–28 mmol/L, pH 7.35–7.45.

What blood gas picture does this represent?

A. Metabolic alkalosis
B. Respiratory acidosis
C. Respiratory alkalosis
D. Type I respiratory failure
E. Type II respiratory failure

2. MANAGING ABDOMINAL PAIN (1)

A 72-year-old woman is brought into hospital with profuse diarrhoea, abdominal pain and fever, which she has suffered for the last two days. On examination, she has generalized abdominal tenderness. Her observations include heart rate 108/min, blood pressure 110/64 mmHg and temperature 38.2°C. Abdominal and erect chest X-rays are unremarkable. Her son tells you she was in hospital two weeks ago with a chest infection.

Which of the following would be the most appropriate treatment in the first instance?

A. Intravenous co-amoxiclav
B. Intravenous vancomycin
C. Oral metronidazole
D. Oral rehydration
E. Subtotal colectomy

3. SHOCK (1)

A 45-year-old man has walked into the emergency department following his involvement in a road traffic collision. On arrival at the hospital he is anxious, but otherwise fine. Later, he suddenly becomes faint. He is taken into the resuscitation room where he is found to have a heart rate of 46/min and a blood pressure of 80/48 mmHg. Primary examination is unremarkable and the patient has warm peripheries.

Which of the following is the most likely cause of his symptoms?

A. Cardiogenic shock
B. Haemorrhagic shock
C. Hypovolaemic shock
D. Neurogenic shock
E. Spinal shock

4. ULCERS (1)

A 53-year-old man presents to the GP with a deep, painful ulcer over the big toe. He gives a 3-month history of severe calf pain on walking which is only eased on resting. Examination shows cool peripheries with reduced distal pulses.

Which ulcer does the patient most likely have?

A. Arterial ulcer
B. Curling ulcer
C. Marjolin ulcer
D. Neuropathic ulcer
E. Venous ulcer

5. PAEDIATRIC SURGERY (1)

A mother brings her 5-week-old son to the paediatric outpatient clinic. She is concerned as he has been having episodes of forceful vomiting after feeds for the last 2 weeks. She says her son always seems hungry and now is beginning to appear lethargic. Examination of the child reveals mild dehydration and the presence of a smooth, firm, non-tender mass in the right upper quadrant of the abdomen. Blood tests are sent.

What biochemical abnormalities would you expect to find?

A. Hyperchloraemic, respiratory alkalosis
B. Hypernatraemic, hyperkalaemic, metabolic alkalosis
C. Hypochloraemic, hyperkalaemic, metabolic alkalosis
D. Hypochloraemic, hypokalaemic, metabolic alkalosis
E. Hyponatraemic, metabolic acidosis

6. PREOPERATIVE MORBIDITY (1)

A 45-year-old woman is due to have an elective cholecystectomy following a recent bout of acute cholecystitis (which has fully resolved). She has a past medical history of high blood pressure, which is fully controlled with tablets.

Which of the following best describes her preoperative morbidity?

A. ASA grade I
B. ASA grade II
C. ASA grade III

D. ASA grade IV

E. ASA grade V

7. UPPER GI BLEED (1)

A 56-year-old man is brought to hospital by his wife. He has been vomiting fresh blood since earlier that morning. She tells you he has a long history of alcohol abuse and drinks at least a bottle of spirits a day.

Which of the following is the most likely cause of his symptoms?

A. Dieulafoy lesions

B. Duodenal ulcer

C. Gastric ulcer

D. Oesophageal varices

E. Oesophagitis

8. LOWER LIMB NERVE LESIONS (1)

A 28-year-old woman was previously admitted to the orthopaedic ward with an ankle fracture which was treated with a plaster cast. When the cast is removed, the patient is unable to dorsiflex her foot. All other leg movements are maintained.

Which nerve has most likely been affected?

A. Common peroneal nerve

B. Obturator nerve

C. Sciatic nerve

D. Sural nerve

E. Tibial nerve

9. BILIARY TRACT DISEASE (1)

A 45-year-old woman presents with a 2-month history of worsening jaundice, itching and malaise. On examination, she has multiple localized areas of yellow pigmentation around her eyes. She has a past history of Sjögren syndrome, but is otherwise well.

What is the most likely diagnosis?

A. Acute cholecystitis

B. Ascending cholangitis

C. Biliary colic

D. Primary biliary cirrhosis

E. Primary sclerosing cholangitis

10. VASCULAR DISEASE (1)

A 28-year-old man presents with a 3-month history of pain in both calves which comes on with walking and is relieved by resting. He is otherwise fit and well, although he does smoke 30 cigarettes a day. On examination, the legs and feet are warm, but the pedal pulses are not palpable. The upper limbs are normal.

What is the most likely diagnosis?

A. Buerger disease
B. Embolus
C. Intermittent claudication
D. Spinal stenosis
E. Takayasu arteritis

11. INVESTIGATING ABDOMINAL PAIN (1)

A 50-year-old woman with known gallstones presents to the emergency department with severe epigastric pain radiating to the back together with nausea and vomiting. Examination reveals localized epigastric peritonitis and investigations reveal an amylase of 650 μ/L.

Which of the following would indicate a poor prognosis in this condition?

A. Amylase of 650 μ/L
B. Arterial pO_2 of 7.0 kPa
C. Patient age of 50 years
D. Pyrexia of 38.5°C
E. White cell count of $10 \times 10^3/\mu L$

12. COMPLICATIONS OF SUPRACONDYLAR FRACTURES

A 6-year-old boy who had a fracture above the left elbow and was treated in a plaster cast is brought into the GP practice by his mother a few days after plaster removal. She is worried due to the abnormal positioning of his forearm. On examination, his left forearm appears to be shortened and held in flexion at the wrist and the fingers.

Which of the following complications has led to this appearance?

A. Brachial artery injury
B. Lack of physiotherapy
C. Malunion at fracture site
D. Median nerve injury
E. Ulnar nerve injury

13. DYSPHAGIA (1)

A 40-year-old man presents to the GP complaining of increasing difficulty in swallowing over the last few months. He tells you he has been working in Mexico for the last two years with a new business. He is otherwise well and denies any other symptoms.

Which of the following is the most likely cause of his symptoms?

A. Chagas disease
B. Gastro-oesophageal reflux disease
C. Myasthenia gravis
D. Plummer-Vinson syndrome
E. Zenker diverticulum

14. BREAST DISEASE (1)

A 30-year-old woman presents with multiple bilateral breast swellings which cause her discomfort, particularly just before her periods. They have been present for several years but appear to be getting worse.

What is the most likely diagnosis?

A. Duct ectasia
B. Fat necrosis
C. Fibroadenoma
D. Fibrocystic disease
E. Peau d'orange

15. SHORTNESS OF BREATH

You are called to see a 56-year-old man who is one day post appendicectomy because he became acutely short of breath. He has just been given his first dose of cyclizine to relieve nausea. On arrival, the patient is breathless with the following observations: heart rate 122/min, blood pressure 86/48 mmHg and saturations 85% in air.

Which of the following would you administer first?

A. Adrenaline
B. Chlorphenamine
C. Fluids
D. Hydrocortisone
E. Salbutamol

16. ABDOMINAL PAIN (1)

A 34 year-old man presents to the emergency department with a 10-hour history of abdominal pain associated with nausea and vomiting. On examination, the patient is lying still and has tenderness with guarding in the right iliac fossa. His temperature is 37.6°C. He has no significant past medical history.

What is the most likely diagnosis?

A. Appendicitis
B. Crohn disease
C. Meckel diverticulitis
D. Mesenteric adenitis
E. Renal colic

17. ENDOCRINE DISEASE (1)

A 43-year-old man presents to the GP with a 2-month history of worsening headaches. The headaches are almost constant and are worse in the morning. On examination, his skin is thick and greasy and he is hypertensive.

What is the most likely diagnosis?

A. Acromegaly
B. Addison disease
C. Congenital adrenal hyperplasia
D. Conn syndrome
E. Phaeochromocytoma

18. JAUNDICE (1)

A 55-year-old man presents to the emergency department with increasing itching and upper abdominal discomfort. His wife has noticed that he is looking 'yellow'. On examination, there is a non-tender mass in the right upper quadrant. The patient has a history of ulcerative colitis, which is currently in remission.
What is the most likely diagnosis?

A. Cholangiocarcinoma
B. Gallstones
C. Haemolysis
D. Hepatitis
E. Pancreatic carcinoma

19. SPINAL CORD LESIONS (1)

A 27-year-old man presents to the emergency department after being stabbed in the back. He is now unable to move his right leg. On examination, you note that he cannot feel pain on the left leg, although motor function in this limb is preserved.
What is the most likely diagnosis?

A. Anterior cord syndrome
B. Brown-Séquard syndrome
C. Central cord syndrome
D. Posterior cord syndrome
E. Syringomyelia

20. HEPATOMEGALY (1)

A 12-year-old boy is brought to the GP practice by his mother with a 2-month history of malaise and a worsening yellowing of his skin. His mother says that he has been behaving differently the last few days. On examination, his abdomen is slightly distended and the liver is palpable.
What is the most likely diagnosis?

A. Haemochromatosis
B. Hepatitis A
C. Infectious mononucleosis
D. Riedel lobe
E. Wilson disease

21. ANORECTAL DISEASE (1)

A 70-year-old woman presents with a 2-month history of anal pain and itching. More recently she had been having some fresh bleeding and mucous discharge per rectum. On examination, there is an irregular tender ulceration at the anal margin which appears to be extending into the anal canal.

What is the most likely diagnosis?

A. Anal carcinoma
B. Anal fissure
C. Anal warts
D. Fistula-in-ano
E. Primary syphilis

22. STATISTICS (1)

A new form of CT scan is being piloted to help detect scaphoid fractures. A study looked at 600 people: 300 people with scaphoid fractures and 300 without. The trial produced 250 positive results and 350 negative results. Of the 250 positive results, there were no false positives, and of the 350 negative results, 50 were false negatives.

What is the sensitivity of CT scanning in detecting scaphoid fractures in this study?

A. 17%
B. 33%
C. 50%
D. 83%
E. 100%

23. HERNIAS (1)

A newborn baby boy is found to have visible intestine emerging from his abdomen. There is no covering to the contents.

Which of the following is the most likely diagnosis?

A. Epigastric hernia
B. Exomphalos
C. Gastroschisis
D. Paraumbilical hernia
E. Umbilical hernia

24. GASTROINTESTINAL POLYPS (1)

A 27-year-old woman is undergoing a routine surveillance colonoscopy for ulcerative colitis. The endoscopist notes multiple small projections throughout the bowel that are of a similar colour to the normal bowel mucosa.

What is the most likely morphology of the polyps?

A. Adenomatous polyp
B. Hamartomatous polyp
C. Juvenile polyp
D. Metaplastic polyp
E. Pseudopolyp

25. FOOT DISORDERS (1)

A 45-year-old woman presents to the orthopaedic clinic with a 6-week history of shooting pains in her right foot, radiating to her toes, only experienced when wearing her shoes. On examination, there is tenderness between the third and fourth metatarsal heads. Foot X-rays are reported as normal.

Which of the following is the most likely diagnosis?

A. Bunion
B. Gout
C. March fracture
D. Morton neuroma
E. Plantar fasciitis

26. GROIN LUMPS (1)

A 69-year-old man presents with a swelling in his right groin. He otherwise feels well. On examination, he has a medial lying, minimally tender pulsatile lump. He tells you he recently suffered from a heart attack and had an angioplasty.

What is the most likely diagnosis?

A. False aneurysm
B. Femoral hernia
C. Groin abscess
D. Inguinal hernia
E. Saphena varix

27. TUMOUR MARKERS (1)

A 65-year-old woman presents with episodes of lower abdominal pain and intermittent vaginal bleeding. On examination, there is a palpable mass in the lower abdomen.

Which of the following tumour markers would be associated with this presentation?

A. Alpha fetoprotein
B. Beta-hCG
C. CA 125
D. Calcitonin
E. Carcinoembryonic antigen

28. NIPPLE DISCHARGE (1)

A 38-year-old woman presents to the GP with pain in the subareolar region of the left breast associated with occasional blood-stained nipple discharge. Apart from being extremely anxious she has no other associated symptoms. Examination is unremarkable.

What is the most likely diagnosis?

A. Duct ectasia
B. Galactocoele
C. Intraductal papilloma
D. Paget disease ·
E. Prolactinoma

29. THYROID DISEASE (1)

A 76-year-old man presents to the GP with a rapidly growing lump in his neck. It is now causing him difficulty swallowing. Examination reveals a 4 cm hard mass in the front of the neck that is fixed to the overlying skin.

What is the most likely diagnosis?

A. Anaplastic carcinoma
B. Follicular carcinoma
C. Graves disease
D. Papillary carcinoma
E. Toxic multinodular goitre

30. ABDOMINAL PAIN (2)

A 27 year old man presents to the emergency department with a 6-hour history of upper abdominal pain radiating to the back and associated vomiting. On examination, he has marked epigastric tenderness and you notice a bluish discolouration around his umbilicus. His heart rate is 118/min and blood pressure is 108/76 mmHg.

Which of the following blood analytes would be most useful in identifying a diagnosis?

A. Amylase
B. C-reactive protein
C. Haemoglobin
D. Sodium
E. Urea

31. INVESTIGATING ENDOCRINE DISEASE (1)

A 32-year-old woman presents to the GP with a 1-month history of panic attacks. She says the attacks are associated with sweating and the feeling of her heart thumping in her chest. She cannot always think of a precipitator to these attacks, but they are increasing in frequency. Examination is unremarkable.

Which of the following investigations will be the most helpful in confirming the diagnosis?

A. 17-hydroxyprogesterone levels
B. 24-hour urinary vanillylmandelic acid
C. 24-hour urinary 5-hydroxyindole acetic acid
D. Serum calcitonin
E. Short synacthen test

32. MANAGING COMMON FRACTURES (1)

A 27-year-old man is brought into the resuscitation room having been hit by a car. The patient is stable and his only injury is a fractured right tibia with overlying tissue loss of around 3 cm. His leg is currently in a splint. His distal pulses are palpable.

What would be the most appropriate next step in management?

A. Dress wound
B. External fixation of fracture
C. Internal fixation of fracture
D. Intravenous antibiotics and debridement of tissue
E. Plaster immobilization of fracture

33. SKIN LESIONS (1)

A 22-year-old woman presents to the GP practice with a scaly, well-defined red rash on her cheeks. She has also noticed its appearance on her scalp. There is some associated hair loss.

What is the most likely diagnosis?

A. Acne vulgaris
B. Discoid lupus
C. Erysipelas
D. Impetigo
E. Rosacea

34. SHOULDER DISORDERS (1)

An 18-year-old boy is brought into the emergency department following an epileptic seizure. On recovery he complains of pain in the right shoulder. Examination reveals the arm to be held adducted and internally rotated with a fullness at the posterior aspect of the shoulder. There is resistance to passive external rotation.

Which of the following injuries is the patient most likely to have sustained?

A. Acromioclavicular dislocation
B. Anterior dislocation of the shoulder
C. Inferior dislocation of the shoulder

D. Posterior dislocation of the shoulder
E. Sternoclavicular dislocation

35. MANAGING VENOUS DISEASE (1)

A 63-year-old woman with known varicose veins presents to the surgical outpatients with a fever and a sloughy shallow ulcer above the medial aspect of the ankle with surrounding cellulitis.
   Which of the following would be the best immediate treatment option?

A. Debridement and intravenous antibiotics
B. Debridement and topical antibiotics
C. Debridement and sclerotherapy
D. Graded compression bandaging
E. Stripping of the long saphenous vein

36. CUTANEOUS MALIGNANCIES (1)

A 60-year-old Asian woman presents to the GP having noticed a dark brown lesion on the palm of her left hand which has been present for 2 months. She initially thought it was a bruise but it has been slowly enlarging.
   What is the most likely diagnosis?

A. Acral lentiginous melanoma
B. Amelanocytic melanoma
C. Lentigo maligna melanoma
D. Nodular melanoma
E. Superficial spreading malignant melanoma

37. NECK LUMPS (1)

A 12-year-old girl is brought to the GP by her mother having noticed a painless swelling on the left side of her neck following a recent cold. On examination, there is a smooth, fluctuant, non-tender swelling anterior to the sternocleidomastoid muscle.
   What is the most likely diagnosis?

A. Branchial cyst
B. Cervical rib
C. Cystic hygroma
D. Sternocleidomastoid tumour
E. Thyroglossal cyst

38. COMPLICATIONS OF NASAL FRACTURE

A 27-year-old man presents to the emergency department complaining of severe nasal pain and a blocked nose. On examination, he has a bluish discoloured swelling over the bridge of the nose. His friend tells you he was assaulted four days ago.

What is the most likely cause of his symptoms?

A. Fracture of the orbit
B. Fracture of the cribriform plate
C. Intranasal foreign body
D. Maxillary sinusitis
E. Septal haematoma

39. MANAGING TESTICULAR PAIN (1)

A 17-year-old boy presents to the emergency department at 1 am with a 3-hour history of pain in his right testicle. He denies any trauma but does a lot of long distance running. Examination is difficult due to pain; however the right testicle does appear to be swollen, slightly red and extremely tender.
Which of the following do you do next?

A. Admit for urgent ultrasound scan the next morning
B. Contact the urologist on call and organize urgent ultrasound scan
C. Contact the urologist on call and prepare for theatre
D. Obtain a urine sample and prescribe antibiotics
E. Prescribe strong analgesia and advise to stop running till symptoms resolve

40. CHEST TRAUMA (1)

A 27-year-old man who was the driver of a car involved in a high speed collision with a truck is brought into the resuscitation room. On arrival, he is complaining of severe left-sided chest pain. You note that he is breathless, tachycardic and hypotensive. He has reduced air entry on the left side of the chest and the trachea is deviated to the right.
What would you do next?

A. Insert a chest drain into the fifth intercostal space
B. Insert a wide bore cannula into the second intercostal space
C. Request an urgent chest X-ray
D. Request an urgent ECG
E. Perform a pericardiocentesis

41. EYE DISEASE (1)

A 54-year-old man presents to the emergency department in the middle of the night with acute pain in his left eye, blurred vision and vomiting. He tells you it happened suddenly while he was watching TV. On examination his cornea is injected and the eyeball feels hard. His pupil is semi-dilated and fixed.
How would you manage this patient in the first instance?

A. Refer patient for iridectomy
B. Topical aciclovir
C. Topical antibiotics

D. Topical pilocarpine
E. Topical steroids

42. PAEDIATRIC ORTHOPAEDICS (1)

A 6-year-old boy is brought into the emergency department by his father with a 1-day history of right hip pain. There is no history of trauma and the child is systemically well. On examination, the child is afebrile and there is generalized reduced range of movement of the hip. Blood tests and X-rays show no abnormality.

What is the most likely diagnosis?

A. Congenital dislocation of the hip
B. Irritable hip
C. Perthes disease
D. Septic arthritis
E. Slipped upper femoral epiphysis

43. INVESTIGATING DYSPHAGIA (1)

A 54-year-old woman presents to the GP complaining of generalized muscle weakness, difficulty swallowing and blurred vision, all of which are worse at the end of the day. Examination is unremarkable apart from ptosis of the right eye.

Which of the following investigations would be most useful in establishing the cause of her symptoms?

A. Creatine kinase levels
B. Electromyography
C. Muscle biopsy
D. Tensilon test
E. Troponin levels

44. INVESTIGATING UROLOGICAL DISEASE (1)

A 72-year-old man comes to see you in the GP practice complaining of a 6-month history of urinary hesitancy, poor stream and occasional incontinence. He is increasingly troubled by his symptoms. Blood test results show a prostate specific antigen of 30 ng/mL.

Which of the following is the most appropriate next step?

A. Antibiotics
B. Medical management with alpha-blockers
C. Referral for transurethral resection of prostate
D. Urgent referral for renal tract ultrasound
E. Urgent referral for transrectal ultrasound and prostate biopsy

45. ABDOMINAL PAIN (3)

A 64-year-old woman presents with a 2-day history of increasing left-sided abdominal pain with fever. On examination, she has localized peritonism in the left iliac fossa. Her blood tests reveal a raised white cell count and C-reactive protein.

What of the following is the most likely diagnosis?

Which of the following is the most likely diagnosis?

A. Constipation
B. Diverticular disease
C. Diverticulitis
D. Diverticulosis
E. Irritable bowel syndrome

46. BONE TUMOURS (1)

A 14-year-old boy who has been complaining of pain and a localized tender swelling above his right knee for a month has been sent for X-rays by his GP. The X-ray shows an ill-defined breach in the lower end of the cortex of the femur with periosteal elevation and calcification.

What is the most likely diagnosis?

A. Chondrosarcoma
B. Ewing sarcoma
C. Lipoma
D. Osteoma
E. Osteosarcoma

47. HAEMATURIA

A 63-year-old man presents to the GP practice following two episodes of passing blood in his urine. These episodes were not associated with pain. He has no past medical history of note but is a lifelong smoker.

Which of the following is the most likely cause?

A. Cystitis
B. Diverticulitis
C. Renal calculi
D. Transitional cell carcinoma
E. Urethral injury

48. THE SWOLLEN LIMB (1)

A 4-week-old baby girl is brought to the paediatrics clinic with swelling of both legs which the parents feel has been present since birth. On examination there is oedema, which is non-pitting and firm to touch, of both lower limbs to the knee.

What is the most likely diagnosis?

A. Elephantiasis
B. Hereditary angioedema
C. Lymphoedema praecox
D. Lymphoedema tarda
E. Milroy disease

49. PAEDIATRIC SURGICAL MANAGEMENT (1)

An 8-year-old boy is brought to the emergency department with a 3-day history of left-sided flank and abdominal pain, fevers and reduced appetite. On examination, he has minimal left-sided flank and lower abdominal tenderness, and there is a fluctuant, non-tender swelling in the child's groin. You note that the child is walking with a limp and there is pain in the hip region on straight leg raising against resistance.

How would this child be best managed?

A. Appendicectomy
B. Arthroscopic hip washout
C. Exploration of testes
D. Incision and drainage with intravenous antibiotics
E. Intravenous antibiotics alone

50. UPPER LIMB PAIN

A 33-year-old woman has been referred to the orthopaedic clinic by her GP. She complains of a 2-month history of pain and numbness in the left hand, which is worse at night, together with difficulty gripping. On examination, there is reduced sensation over the thumb, index and middle finger together with some wasting of the thenar eminence and weakness of thumb abduction. Her symptoms can be recreated by forcibly bending the wrist.

Compression of which of the following structures is resulting in her symptoms?

A. Median nerve
B. Radial artery
C. Radial nerve
D. Ulnar artery
E. Ulnar nerve

Practice Paper 1: Answers

1. ARTERIAL BLOOD GASES (1)

D – Type I respiratory failure

A simple interpretation of arterial blood gases is as follows. The pH value shows if the gas is acidotic (<7.35) or alkalotic (>7.45). Next you need to find out if the alkalosis or acidosis is due to a metabolic or respiratory cause – this is done by looking at the pCO_2 and bicarbonate levels. There are two things you need to bear in mind before continuing: (1) carbon dioxide is acidic and bicarbonate is alkaline; and (2) bicarbonate equates to 'metabolic' and pCO_2 means 'respiratory'. An alkalosis can be due to either a high bicarbonate ('metabolic alkalosis') or a low pCO_2 ('respiratory alkalosis'). Conversely, an acidosis can be caused by either a low bicarbonate ('metabolic acidosis') or a high pCO_2 ('respiratory acidosis').

In some cases of blood gas disturbance the body has time to compensate. In other words, whichever chemical is causing the imbalance is counteracted by the opposite one. For example, if there is a high bicarbonate (metabolic alkalosis) then the pCO_2 starts to increase to bring in some acidity and counteract the alkalosis. This is achieved by 'under breathing', leading to relative retention of CO_2.

If compensation is successful the pH will return to within the normal range (7.35–7.45), even if the bicarbonate and pCO_2 levels are abnormal. It is important to know that the body cannot *over*compensate, i.e. if there is an initial acidosis, the body will not make that into an alkalosis, and the pH will always remain on the acidic side of normal (<7.40). Similarly a compensated alkalosis will always have a pH > 7.40, the alkalotic side of normal.

Respiratory failure is defined as a pO_2 < 8.0. Type I respiratory failure occurs when there is hypoxia in the presence of a low or normal pCO_2. Type II respiratory failure is hypoxia in the presence of a high pCO_2.

The pH, pCO_2 and bicarbonate levels are normal in this case, so there is no acid-base disorder. However this man has a hypoxia (pO_2 < 8) which denotes respiratory failure. Because the pCO_2 is not high, it is a type I respiratory failure. This man's hypoxia is probably secondary to a chest infection.

2. MANAGING ABDOMINAL PAIN (1)

C – Oral metronidazole

This patient has presented with the features of pseudomembranous colitis. Pseudomembranous colitis is an acute inflammatory condition which occurs secondary to antibiotic use. The majority of cases are caused by an overgrowth of the Gram-positive anaerobe *Clostridium difficile,* following a change in the normal bacterial flora of the gut secondary to antibiotic use. Clindamycin, ampicillin, cephalosporins and ciprofloxacin are common responsible agents, although almost any antibiotic can be the cause. Presentation is usually within 3 to 9 days, although symptoms may develop up to 6 weeks after antibiotic use. Patients present with profuse offensive diarrhoea, abdominal pain and constitutional symptoms, such as fever and malaise. Twenty percent of cases are localized to the proximal colon and caecum and present with a right lower quadrant pain which may mimic appendicitis. Blood tests often reveal a raised white cell count. The diagnosis is established on stool testing for *C. difficile* toxins. A 'pseudomembrane' (patches of infective debris) may be seen in the rectum and colon (although endoscopy is now rarely performed).

Treatment involves adequate fluid resuscitation (mild cases do not require admission) and administration of oral metronidazole for 10 days. Resistant and recurrent cases are treated with oral vancomycin (intravenous preparations are avoided as the drug does not reach the intestinal mucosa). Anti-diarrhoeal agents must be avoided as this would lead to retention of the *C. difficile* toxin.

Complications of pseudomembranous colitis include hypovolaemic shock, electrolyte imbalance, hypoalbuminaemia, perforation of the bowel and toxic megacolon. Patients who develop toxic megacolon require surgery to remove the affected segment of bowel (subtotal colectomy). Toxic megacolon appears as a dilated colon with a featureless wall on plain abdominal X-ray.

A fifth of patients who have been successfully treated for pseudomembranous colitis have a relapse. Pseudomembranous colitis is a common hospital acquired infection (spread by the faeco-oral route) and highlights the importance of good hygiene and hand washing.

Clostridium, from Greek *kloster* = spindle (pertaining to the bacterium's rod-like shape).

3. SHOCK (1)

D – Neurogenic shock

Neurogenic shock is caused by sudden disruption or injury to the sympathetic nervous pathways, resulting in the loss of vasomotor tone and pooling of blood in the peripheries. This leads to profound hypotension.

Unlike most forms of shock, neurogenic shock is also characterized by bradycardia. Causes of neurogenic shock include injury to the brain and spinal cord, and acute emotional stress.

Neurogenic shock must be differentiated from spinal shock. *Spinal shock* is a transient state occurring after injury to the spinal cord. There is loss of all voluntary and reflex activity below the level of the injury, resulting in a hypotonic flaccid paralysis which also affects the bladder and bowel. This loss can be complete initially but may resolve over a period of days and weeks following the injury.

Stabilizing the spine is crucial in the resuscitation of these patients. *Haemorrhagic shock* is a form of hypovolaemic shock, in which blood loss is too great to maintain an effective circulating volume. The cause is usually acute and is treated by replacing lost fluid/blood, identifying the source of blood loss and preventing further bleeding. *Cardiogenic shock* is defined as hypotension with tissue hypoperfusion despite adequate ventricular filling. In essence, it occurs from a failure of the heart to act as an effective pump. Cardiogenic shock most commonly occurs following myocardial infarction. Other causes include arrhythmias and valvular abnormalities. Examination may reveal signs of heart failure, such as an elevated jugular venous pressure (JVP) and pulmonary/pedal oedema.

4. ULCERS (1)

A – Arterial ulcer

Arterial ulcers are typically painful, deep, well demarcated and occur on the heels, toes and over bony prominences. They occur as a result of arterial insufficiency and ischaemia, the most common cause of this being atherosclerosis. This patient has symptoms of intermittent claudication, which together with poor pulses would suggest an arterial cause of the ulcer. Other findings which would suggest an ischaemic ulcer include a dusky discolouration with shiny, hairless skin and thickening of the toenails. Contrast angiography will help define arterial lesions which may be improved by angioplasty or vascular reconstruction.

Venous ulcers are most common in women after middle age. They are caused by venous hypertension and are commonly associated with varicose veins. They typically appear over the medial gaiter area (from the ankle to the proximal calf) and are shallow and sloughy. Surrounding skin may be oedematous, dark (caused by haemosiderin deposition), eczematous and thickened (lipodermatosclerosis).

When taking a history from a 'vascular patient' be sure to cover the vascular risk factors such as a personal or family history of diabetes, smoking habits and exertional capacity before onset of claudication (e.g. walking distance, number of stairs they can climb).

5. PAEDIATRIC SURGERY (1)

D – Hypochloraemic, hypokalaemic, metabolic alkalosis
This patient has presented with the symptoms and signs of pyloric stenosis, caused by hypertrophy and hyperplasia of the muscle layers of the pylorus. It is the most common cause of mechanical obstruction in children, with an incidence of up to 4/1000. It is four times as common in male infants (30% of these being the first born) and can present anywhere between the first and eighteenth week of life, but commonly presents 6–8 weeks after birth. It is characterized by non-bilious, projectile vomiting. Diagnosis is confirmed by the presence of an 'olive' shaped mass in the right upper quadrant, usually post vomit or when the child is relaxed. It can also be confirmed by ultrasound examination. Due to the loss of gastric fluid, there is a hypochloraemic metabolic alkalosis. Renal exchange of potassium for hydrogen (a compensatory mechanism) leads to hypokalaemia. Dehydration can result in either hypo- or hypernatraemia. Treatment initially consists of fluid and electrolyte resuscitation followed by definitive treatment in the form of surgery (Ramstedt pyloromyotomy, where the pyloric muscle is divided longitudinally down to the mucosal layer). The baby can tolerate milk feeds a few hours after the operation.

6. PREOPERATIVE MORBIDITY (1)

B – ASA grade II
The American Society of Anesthesiologists (ASA) grading system is the most commonly used scale to predict a patient's preoperative morbidity irrespective of the surgery they are about to undergo. Patients are assigned a preoperative grade according to the following scale:

Grade I   = normal, healthy individual (0.05% anaesthetic mortality)
Grade II   = mild systemic disease that does not limit activity (0.4% mortality)
Grade III   = severe systemic disease that limits activity but is not incapacitating (4.5% mortality)
Grade IV   = incapacitating systemic disease that is constantly life-threatening (25% mortality)
Grade V   = moribund, not expected to survive over 24 hours with or without surgery (50% mortality)

In addition to the above grading scale, an 'E' suffix is used to denote an emergency operation.

7. UPPER GI BLEED (1)

D – Oesophageal varices
This patient has presented with haematemesis; vomiting fresh blood from the upper gastrointestinal tract. From the history, this patient has most

likely developed liver cirrhosis and, as a result, oesophageal varices secondary to portal hypertension. Portal hypertension results in the formation of collateral vessels between the portal and systemic circulations as follows:

- Left gastric and oesophageal veins (→ oesophageal and gastric varices)
- Obliterated umbilical vein to the superior and inferior epigastric veins (→ caput medusae)
- Superior and inferior rectal veins (→ anal canal varices)
- Retroperitoneum

Other features of portal hypertension are splenomegaly and ascites. The management of variceal bleeding is by immediate resuscitation followed by an urgent endoscopy to identify and control the bleeding.

Inflammation of the oesophagus (oesophagitis) is largely caused by gastro-oesophageal reflux disease (GORD), where failure of relaxation of the lower oesophageal sphincter allows the reflux of stomach contents back into the oesophagus. Symptoms include retrosternal chest pain and cough. Longstanding GORD is a risk factor for developing adenocarcinoma of the oesophagus. A Dieulafoy lesion is an abnormally tortuous, large-calibre, submucosal artery. It is found in 5% of the population and in 95% of cases occurs on the lesser curvature of the stomach, 6 cm away from the gastro-oesophageal junction. Lesions are largely asymptomatic until they bleed.

Paul Georges Dieulafoy, French surgeon (1839–1911).

8. LOWER LIMB NERVE LESIONS (1)

A – Common peroneal nerve

The common peroneal nerve (or common fibular nerve) is a branch of the sciatic nerve which supplies the dorsiflexors and evertor muscles of the foot and sensation to the lateral lower leg and upper foot. The common peroneal nerve lies in close proximity to the head of the fibula and may become trapped by below-knee plaster casts or damaged with fibular fractures. Features of common peroneal nerve lesions include lack of dorsiflexion (with a resulting foot drop) and loss of sensation in the anterolateral lower leg and dorsum of the foot (except for the lateral aspect of the foot which is supplied by the sural nerve). The inability to dorsiflex the foot will result in a 'foot drop' with a 'high-stepping' gait to ensure it is not scraped along the ground.

Peroneal, from Greek *perone* = pin (describing the shape of the fibula).

9. BILIARY TRACT DISEASE (1)

D – Primary biliary cirrhosis

Primary biliary cirrhosis is an autoimmune condition that commonly affects middle-aged women. It is characterized by inflammation and fibrosis of the bile canaliculi, resulting in cholestasis. The majority of cases are associated with rheumatoid arthritis and Sjögren syndrome (characterized by dry eyes – xerophthalmia – and a dry mouth – xerostomia). Common presenting symptoms are described above and include xanthelasmata (cholesterol deposits around the eyes) but patients may also present with the complications of liver cirrhosis and portal hypertension. Tests for anti-mitochondrial antibody are usually positive, but a definitive diagnosis is made on liver biopsy. Treatment is aimed at reducing cholestasis and promoting the excretion of bile salts. The development of primary biliary cirrhosis is an indication for a liver transplant, although the condition can recur in the transplanted organ.

Primary sclerosing cholangitis is an autoimmune inflammatory condition characterized by chronic fibrosis of both the intra- and extra-hepatic biliary tree. It is most common in middle-aged men and has an increased incidence in those with ulcerative colitis (70%), HIV and retroperitoneal fibrosis. Patients present with jaundice, intermittent fevers, pruritus and right upper quadrant pain. Diagnosis is confirmed on ERCP, which will show 'beading' of the biliary tree upon retrograde injection of contrast (a result of intermittent stricture formation). Definitive management is with a liver transplant. Primary sclerosing cholangitis is a risk factor for developing cholangiocarcinoma (affects at least 10%).

Acute cholecystitis is an inflammation of the gallbladder most commonly arising secondary to a blockage of biliary outflow by a gallstone in the cystic duct or stone impaction in Hartmann pouch (an anatomical area at the neck of the gallbladder where stones commonly become trapped). Collections of fluid that are not able to 'flow' due to blockage commonly become infected.

Ascending cholangitis refers to a condition where biliary stasis occurs due to a downstream obstruction (commonly a stone, stricture or malignancy) which, again, causes stasis of fluid which can become infected. This can cause profound sepsis and one must seek to resuscitate the patient and relieve the obstruction. This can be done via ERCP (stenting for stricture or balloon trawl for stones) or percutaneous drainage of the biliary system.

Greek *xērós* = dry.

10. VASCULAR DISEASE (1)

A – Buerger disease

Buerger disease is a vasculitis of medium-sized vessels that results in progressive obliteration of distal arteries in young men (<45 years) who smoke heavily. It is most common in Asians and Ashkenazi Jews, and is associated with HLA-B$_{12}$. Buerger disease affects the upper and lower limbs. The main symptom is pain, but chronic inflammation and thrombosis can result in ulceration and gangrene, often requiring amputations.

Arteriography shows normal proximal vessels and distal occlusions with multiple 'corkscrew' collaterals. Management is with analgesia and stopping smoking. If tobacco use is not ceased, multiple amputations will be unavoidable.

Takayasu arteritis (a.k.a. pulseless disease or aortic-arch syndrome) is a rare vasculitis characterized by granulomatous inflammation of the aorta and its major branches. Features include hypertension, arm claudication, absent pulses, bruits and visual disturbance (transient amblyopia and blindness). Patients also present with systemic illness (malaise, fever, night sweats and weight loss). It is most common in younger Asian women. Diagnosis is by angiography which shows narrowing of the aorta and its major branches. Management is with steroids but the condition is progressive and death occurs within a few years.

Leo Buerger, Austrian-born American physician and urologist (1879–1943).

Mikito Takayasu, Japanese ophthalmologist (1860–1938).

11. INVESTIGATING ABDOMINAL PAIN (1)

B – Arterial pO$_2$ of 7.0 kPa

Pancreatitis is inflammation of the pancreas confirmed by a raised amylase (above four times the normal upper limit) or elevated serum lipase (twice the upper normal limit). Biliary disease and alcohol account for up to 80% of cases, with 10% being a combination of these. A significant proportion of cases are idiopathic.

The features below, according to the modified Glasgow criteria, are markers of a poor prognosis. Patients should be scored on admission according to:

Age	> 55 years
White cell count	> 15 × 10^3/μL
Urea	> 16 mmol/L
Glucose	> 10 mmol/L
Arterial pO$_2$	< 8 kPa
Albumin	< 32 mmol/L
Calcium	< 2.0 mmol/L
Lactate dehydrogenase	> 600 mmol/L

The mnemonic PANCREAS can be used to remember the modified Glasgow criteria: pO$_2$, Age, Neutrophils (WCC), Calcium, Renal (urea), Enzymes (LDH, AST), Albumin, Sugar (glucose).

Severe disease is present if three or more of the criteria are present within 48 hours. Note that the prognosis is unaltered by the serum amylase concentration. Other prognostic scores for acute pancreatitis are the Ranson's criteria and APACHE II.

For more details on pancreatitis, see the question 'Abdominal pain (2)'.

12. COMPLICATIONS OF SUPRACONDYLAR FRACTURES

A – Brachial artery injury

This boy has presented with Volkmann ischaemic contracture, a flexion contracture of the hand and wrist, caused by circulatory compromise and ischaemia leading to fibrosis of the forearm compartment. It is a recognized complication of supracondylar fractures, secondary to untreated compartment syndrome (which in this case is likely to have been from a simultaneous brachial artery injury or occlusion). Other recognized complications of supracondylar fractures are median nerve injury, anywhere along its course from the elbow down, usually resulting in carpal tunnel syndrome, and stretching of the ulnar nerve over an increasing valgus deformity, causing ulnar nerve palsy as the child grows (tardy ulnar nerve palsy). Malunion of supracondylar fractures leads to a cubitus varus deformity ('gunstock deformity'). Treatment of Volkmann ischaemic contracture involves surgery to release the contracted muscles.

Richard von Volkmann, German surgeon (1830–1889).

13. DYSPHAGIA (1)

A – Chagas disease

Chagas disease is a parasitic disease of the tropics caused by the protozoan *Trypanosoma cruzi*. Transmission can be vector borne, via blood transfusion and the placenta. Chagas disease is endemic to Central America and South America. Symptoms depend on the stage of infection. In the acute stages, a skin nodule – a chagoma – appears at the site of inoculation (it may go unnoticed) and is associated with non-specific symptoms such as fevers, malaise, anorexia and lymphadenopathy. These symptoms usually resolve spontaneously. The second stage in Chagas disease may occur after many years (and affects around 30%). One common presenting complaint is dysphagia, caused by the destruction of the oesophageal myenteric plexus with subsequent disruption of peristalsis. The retained food eventually results in oesophageal dilatation, and a 'megaoesophagus' can be seen on barium swallow. Other secondary features of Chagas disease include cardiomyopathy and dementia. Treatment is with a combination of anti-parasitic medication and by the management of clinical manifestations. Presenting features of Chagas disease are similar to those experienced in oesophageal achalasia, an idiopathic condition caused by the degeneration of Auerbach plexus (see the question, 'Managing dysphagia').

It is thought that Charles Darwin had contracted, and eventually died from, Chagas disease.

Carlos Chagas, Brazilian physician (1879–1934).

14. BREAST DISEASE (1)

D – Fibrocystic disease

Fibrocystic disease of the breast is a common benign condition affecting more than half of women, commonly between the ages of 30 and 50. The main pathological abnormalities are small cyst formation, fibrosis and hyperplasia of the duct epithelium. It is characterized by nodular changes in breast tissue and may be considered a normal variant. Symptoms are variable from aching to severe breast pain (mastalgia), typically eased following menstruation, and itching of the nipples. Treatment is largely symptomatic, although larger cysts may be aspirated (such cysts can often recur following aspiration). Regular self-examination is important so as not to overlook any co-existing cancerous breast disease.

Fat necrosis is most common in obese, middle-aged women with a history of trauma to the area. It presents with a painless, irregular, firm lump in the breast and may be associated with skin thickening or retraction. The size of the lump usually decreases in size with time but may leave residual fat cysts within the breast. The diagnosis of fat necrosis must be confirmed by core biopsy as the presenting features may be similar to those of carcinoma.

Peau d'orange is the term used to describe the orange-peel appearance of oedematous, dimpled skin that occurs when there is malignant infiltration from underlying breast cancer preventing normal lymphatic drainage.

15. SHORTNESS OF BREATH

A – Adrenaline

This patient is in anaphylactic shock, an acute life-threatening emergency which can rapidly cause death if untreated. Anaphylaxis is a systemic form of the type 1 hypersensitivity reaction, in which exposure to an allergen results in IgE-mediated secretion of inflammatory mediators, such as histamine and prostaglandins, with subsequent vasodilatation and bronchial smooth muscle contraction. This manifests in hypotensive shock and bronchospasm, leading to difficulty breathing, wheezing and pulmonary oedema. Other symptoms include urticaria, angioedema, abdominal pain and diarrhoea. Adrenaline is the primary treatment for anaphylaxis; it acts to bronchodilate and vasoconstrict, and is generally given intramuscularly (10 mL of 1:1000 solution) in this scenario. It has a rapid rate of onset and doses may be repeated. Intravenous antihistamines (e.g. chlorphenamine) and intravenous hydrocortisone are used to assist in dampening the inflammatory response. Fluids are used for hypotension and salbutamol can be administered simultaneously to aid the relief of bronchospasm. Poor response to treatment is an indication for anaesthetic review and possible transfer to an intensive care setting.

Patients who are at risk of anaphylactic shock from common allergens often carry an EpiPen – a preloaded syringe which contains adrenaline for self-administration.

16. ABDOMINAL PAIN (1)

A – Appendicitis

Appendicitis is inflammation of the appendix occurring secondary to obstruction of the appendiceal opening into the caecum. Causes of obstruction include faecoliths and lymphoid hyperplasia secondary to viral infections. Appendicitis is a common cause of an acute abdomen, affecting up to 8% of the population at some point in their life. It is most commonly seen in children and young adults although the mortality associated with appendicitis is greatest at the extremes of age.

The typical presenting features are abdominal pain, which is initially periumbilical and moves to the right iliac fossa, associated with nausea, vomiting and a low grade fever. Diagnosis is largely clinical. Classically there will be localized peritonitis over McBurney point (found one third of the way between the anterior superior iliac spine and umbilicus). Palpation over the left iliac fossa may cause pain in the right iliac fossa (Rovsing sign). An inflamed appendix which lies close to the bladder may present with urinary frequency, one which is close to the rectum with diarrhoea, and if it lies on the psoas muscle the patient will feel most comfortable lying with the hip flexed. The treatment of appendicitis is with appendicectomy. An inflamed appendix which is not removed will become gangrenous and perforate. More rarely, an appendix abscess may develop.

Meckel diverticulitis is inflammation of a Meckel diverticulum (found in 2% of the population). If in a suspected case of appendicitis the appendix appears normal, a Meckel diverticulum must be looked for. An attack of Crohn terminal ileitis presents with right iliac fossa pain. There is a risk of fistula formation when performing an appendicectomy in a patient with Crohn disease. Renal colic typically presents with spasmodic pain which radiates from 'loin to groin' on the affected side, causing the patient to writhe in pain. Stones in the mid-ureter may present with lower abdominal pain, mimicking appendicitis on the right. Mesenteric adenitis is a common cause of right iliac fossa pain in children. This is a transient inflammation of intra-abdominal lymph nodes, often due to a self-limiting viral infection.

Charles McBurney, American surgeon (1845–1913).

Niels Thorkild Rovsing, Danish surgeon (1862–1927).

17. ENDOCRINE DISEASE (1)

A – Acromegaly

The headache is characteristic of an intracranial space-occupying lesion. This, along with the features of greasy skin and hypertension, suggests acromegaly as the most likely cause from the given list. Acromegaly is caused by a growth hormone-secreting tumour of the anterior pituitary gland. The functions of growth hormone include lipolysis, protein synthesis and gluco-neogenesis – in other words it is anabolic. Patients with acromegaly may present with headaches, excessive sweating, thick/oily skin, hypertrophy of soft tissues (large nose/lips/tongue, 'spade-like' hands), big viscera, prognathism (protruding lower jaw) and prominent supraorbital ridges. Other associations are carpal tunnel syndrome, diabetes and hypertension. The pituitary mass may result in features of a space-occupying lesion in the brain, i.e. an early morning headache that is worse on coughing and straining. If a growth hormone-secreting tumour occurs in children before the bone epiphyses have fused, the long bones grow rapidly and gigantism results.

It is important to treat acromegaly because it is associated with an increased risk of atheromatous disease and colon cancer. The diagnosis is made by measuring growth hormone (GH) levels before and after a 75 g glucose load (an oral glucose tolerance test). Glucose normally suppresses GH secretion, but in acromegaly the glucose load has little effect, indicating the autoregulatory negative feedback system is not working correctly and that autonomous GH secretion is occurring. Surgical treatment is by transsphenoid surgery. Medical therapy is with somatostatin analogues (such as intramuscular octreotide) which inhibit GH secretion.

Acromegaly, from Greek *akros* = extremity + *megalos* = large.

18. JAUNDICE (1)

A – Cholangiocarcinoma

This patient has jaundice with a right upper quadrant mass. Courvoisier's law suggests that in the presence of jaundice an enlarged gallbladder is not due to gallstones, as a gallbladder with stones is chronically fibrosed and therefore incapable of enlargement. The finding of this mass is more suggestive of malignancy either in the pancreas or the biliary tree. Cholangiocarcinoma is an adenocarcinoma of the biliary tree and is associated with ulcerative colitis, primary sclerosing cholangitis and to a lesser extent Crohn disease. It usually presents between the ages of 50 and 70 with an equal incidence in men and women. Cholangiocarcinoma has a poor prognosis with an average survival of 6 months, as most are not amenable to curative resection at the time of presentation.

19. SPINAL CORD LESIONS (1)

B – Brown-Séquard syndrome

Brown-Séquard syndrome describes the features of unilateral transection (hemisection) of the spinal cord. Affected patients suffer ipsilateral loss of motor function with impaired joint position and vibration sense (dorsal column dysfunction). There is also a contralateral sensory loss for pain and temperature. This pattern occurs because motor fibres decussate in the medulla to enter the corticospinal tract and sensory fibres for pain and temperature decussate at the level of entry into the spinal cord, resulting in a deficit on the opposite side to the lesion. Brown-Séquard syndrome has the best prognosis of all spinal cord lesions.

Charles-Edouard Brown-Séquard, British neurologist (1817–1894).

20. HEPATOMEGALY (1)

E – Wilson disease

Wilson disease is a rare autosomal recessive condition in which there is a deficiency of caeruloplasmin (a protein involved in the transport of copper), leading to the abnormal deposition of copper in the liver, basal ganglia, eye and other organs. It typically presents in children and young adults with features of liver cirrhosis, neurological disturbance (e.g. gait disturbance, tremor, dysarthria) and psychiatric disturbance (such as emotional lability – present in 15%). Other rarer presentations include renal failure (Fanconi syndrome) and cardiomyopathy. The appearance of copper deposition around the iris is known as Kayser–Fleischer rings and is apparent in 90% of patients with Wilson disease. The diagnosis is made by detecting abnormally low levels of caeruloplasmin, with elevated levels of free copper in the serum, urine and on liver biopsy. Treatment is with penicillamine, which chelates copper and encourages its excretion.

Haemochromatosis is an autosomal recessive disorder of increased dietary absorption of iron. Most cases affect Irish males over 40 years of age. There is systemic iron deposition, for example in the liver (cirrhosis), pancreas (diabetes), heart (cardiac failure) and skin (tanned appearance). The diagnosis is confirmed by liver biopsy, which shows iron deposition with liver fibrosis and cirrhosis. Treatment is by weekly venesection.

Infectious mononucleosis (glandular fever) is a self-limiting illness caused by Epstein–Barr virus. It is most common in teenagers and young adults, and presents with malaise, fevers, sore throat and lymphadenopathy. Hepatosplenomegaly may be found on examination. Treatment is symptomatic. Remember that ampicillin and amoxicillin must not be given to anyone suspected of having infectious mononucleosis as they can precipitate a widespread rash.

Bruno Fleischer, German ophthalmologist (1874–1965).

Bernhard Kayser, German ophthalmologist (1869–1954).

Samuel Alexander Kinnier Wilson, British neurologist (1878–1937).

21. ANORECTAL DISEASE (1)

A – Anal carcinoma

Anal carcinomas account for up to 5% of anorectal malignancies and their incidence is increasing. Anal carcinomas are largely squamous cell carcinomas (80%) unlike their rectal or colonic counterparts which are primarily adenomatous. They occur more commonly in the elderly population and are associated with the human papilloma virus (types 16, 18, 31 and 33) and anal warts. They can also arise within chronic benign lesions, e.g. anal fistulas and haemorrhoids, as a result of recurrent inflammation. The symptoms of anal carcinoma may initially be non-specific, including pain, discomfort, itching, intermittent bleeding and inguinal lymphadenopathy, and as a result it is a diagnosis which may easily be missed in the early stages, particularly as many patients may not have a palpable lesion. Diagnosis is by biopsy and rectal examination under anaesthesia, and CT/MRI can be used to assess the extent of pelvic spread. Localized carcinomas can be treated with radiotherapy with or without excision. Larger tumours may require an abdominoperineal ('AP') resection with colostomy. Here the sigmoid colon, rectum and anus are removed and the defect in the perineum is closed with a mesh or muscle flap.

22. STATISTICS (1)

D – 83%

The *sensitivity* of an investigation is its ability to detect a truly positive result. It is calculated as follows:

$$\text{Sensitivity} = \text{number of true positives}/(\text{number of true positives} + \text{number of false negatives}) \times 100$$

In this case

$$\text{Sensitivity} = 250/(250 + 50) \times 100 = 5/6 \times 100 \approx 83\%$$

Other important definitions in medical statistics include:

The *specificity* is the ability of an investigation to detect a truly negative test result.

$$\text{Specificity} = \text{number of true negatives}/(\text{number of true negatives} + \text{number of false positives}) \times 100$$

The *positive predictive value* (PPV) describes the probability that a condition can be confirmed given a positive test result.

$$\text{PPV} = (\text{number of true positives}/\text{total number of positives}) \times 100$$

The *negative predictive value* (NPV) describes the probability that a condition can be ruled out given a negative test result.

$$\text{NPV} = (\text{number of true negatives}/\text{total number of negatives}) \times 100$$

The *likelihood ratio* is the likelihood that a given test result will be positive in a patient with a certain disorder compared to the likelihood that the same positive result would be expected in a patient without that disorder.

$$\text{Likelihood ratio} = \text{sensitivity}/(1 - \text{specificity})$$

23. HERNIAS (1)

C – Gastroschisis

Gastroschisis is a congenital defect in the anterior abdominal wall adjacent to the umbilicus. Abdominal contents, such as the liver and intestines, can herniated through this defect, but there is no sac covering the contents. Management of gastroschisis is by immediately covering the exposed viscera with clingfilm, followed by operative repair. Gastroschisis is rarely associated with other congenital malformations

Exomphalos is a similar congenital abdominal wall defect where contents of the gut, such as the intestines and liver, lie outside of the body protruding through the umbilicus. These organs lie within a sac made of two membranes – the inner being the peritoneum and the outer being the amniotic membrane. This sac is known as an 'omphalocele'. Treatment is by operative closure. Fifty percent of cases of exomphalos are associated with other congenital malformations, such as trisomies and cardiac defects.

The *umbilical hernia* of infants describes an asymptomatic herniation through a weak umbilicus that develops early in life. It is more common in Afro-Caribbean babies and increases in size on crying. Most umbilical hernias resolve in the first two years of life, but surgery is indicated if it persists beyond this. *Paraumbilical hernias* occur in adults, with herniation through the linea alba just above or below the umbilicus. (The linea alba is a fibrous median line formed by the fusion of anterior and posterior walls of the rectus sheath. This line allows a technically 'bloodless' plane of access to the abdomen during abdominal surgery.) Paraumbilical hernias are much commoner in multiparous women, and as they become large, have a tendency to sag down. Strangulation is a common complication as paraumbilical hernias have narrow necks.

Gastroschisis, from Greek *gastro* = belly + *schisis* = a split.
Linea alba, from Latin *linea* = line + *alba* = white.
Omphalocele, from Greek *omphalos* = navel + *cele* = hernia.
Rectus abdominis, from Latin *rectus* = straight + *abdominus* = abdomen.

24. GASTROINTESTINAL POLYPS (1)

E – Pseudopolyp

Pseudopolyps are found with inflammatory bowel disease. In an area of oedematous, swollen bowel surrounded by ulcerations, it looks as if the oedema is protruding from the walls of the bowel wall as a polyp. In reality, these 'polyps' are merely areas of swollen bowel mucosa.

Juvenile polyps affect 1% of children and young adolescents. They look like a cherry on a stalk. Juvenile polyps are always benign. Some juvenile polyps present with painless bleeding per rectum and can prolapse on defaecation.

Metaplastic polyps are small and usually do not grow to more than 5 mm. Despite the name, they have very little risk of becoming malignant.

25. FOOT DISORDERS (1)

D – Morton neuroma

Morton neuroma is a neuroma of the digital nerve of the foot that is most common between the third and fourth metatarsals. It is a common cause of foot pain and typically presents in women from the age of 40. The pain often occurs on wearing shoes and is relieved when these are removed. Diagnosis is largely clinical but both ultrasound and MRI can confirm the diagnosis. Surgical excision of the neuroma is curative.

Plantar fasciitis causes pain in the heels when walking and results from inflammation of the fascia as it inserts into the calcaneum. *Hallux valgus* is a lateral deviation of the great toe which is relatively common in women past middle age. It is caused by the toe being persistently forced laterally by wearing narrow shoes. Over several years, bunions (a thick-walled bursa) and osteoarthritis can develop over the metatarsal head. Surgical intervention is required in severe cases.

Bunion, from Latin *bunio* = turnip.

Hallux, from Latin *hallux* = great toe.

Thomas Morton, American surgeon (1835–1903).

26. GROIN LUMPS (1)

A – False aneurysm

A false aneurysm (or pseudoaneurysm) is a collection of blood which lies outside of, but communicates with, a vessel. It is held by the surrounding connective tissue and structures. Unlike a true aneurysm, it does not include the vessel wall. False aneurysms commonly follow trauma and iatrogenic injury. False aneurysm formation is a recognized complication of angiography and may be treated by ultrasound-guided compression, embolization or surgery. Infection is another complication of angiography and can present with a groin abscess. Groin abscesses are typically tender and fluctuant but not pulsatile, unless a false aneurysm has become infected.

27. TUMOUR MARKERS (1)

C – CA 125

This patient presents with the symptoms and signs of ovarian carcinoma, which is associated with the tumour marker CA 125 (CA = cancer antigen). Elevated CA 125 levels are not diagnostic but would suggest that further investigation is required if there is a suspicion of ovarian cancer. It is elevated in other malignancies, including endometrial and breast cancers, as well as some benign conditions, such as endometriosis. CA 125 is most useful in assessing response to treatment and predicting recurrence. Another tumour marker associated with ovarian carcinoma is placental alkaline phosphatase.

Carcinoembryonic antigen (CEA) is useful in screening for colorectal cancers and in monitoring response to treatment. Calcitonin is produced by the C-cells of the thyroid gland and elevated levels are associated with medullary thyroid cancers. Beta-hCG (human chorionic gonadotrophin) is a hormone produced by the placenta and therefore is not normally found in men; its presence is associated with testicular tumours. Beta-hCG is also elevated in choriocarcinomas in women and is useful in detecting residual or recurrent disease after treatment. Alpha fetoproteins are produced by the liver and yolk sac of the fetus and levels in adults are normally negligible. Elevated levels are associated with hepatocellular carcinoma and testicular tumours.

A useful list of tumour markers is as follows:

Alpha-fetoprotein	→	hepatocellular carcinoma, testicular tumours
Beta-hCG	→	choriocarcinoma, testicular tumours
CA 125	→	ovarian carcinoma
CA 15-3	→	breast cancer
CA 19-9	→	pancreatic cancer, biliary tract malignancy
Calcitonin	→	medullary thyroid cancer
Carcinoembryonic antigen	→	colorectal tumours
Monoclonal IgG (paraprotein)	→	multiple myeloma
Neurone specific enolase	→	small cell lung cancer
Placental alkaline phosphatase	→	ovarian carcinoma, testicular tumours
Prostate specific antigen	→	prostate cancer
S-100	→	malignant melanoma
Thyroglobulin	→	thyroid tumours

28. NIPPLE DISCHARGE (1)

C – Intraductal papilloma

Intraductal papillomas are benign tumours of the lactiferous glands that usually occur in pre-menopausal women. They commonly present with pain within the nipple or areola, associated with discharge which may be blood-stained. In most cases there is no associated breast lump. Papillomas may be bilateral or multiple, occur more commonly in the younger patient, and are associated with an increased risk of breast carcinoma. Investigation includes cytology, where no malignant cells would be found; ultrasound, which is more sensitive than mammography for intraductal papillomas; and ductography. If a lump is present, a biopsy can also be taken. Treatment can be conservative but if there are significant symptoms or a risk of malignancy then surgical excision of the affected duct can be undertaken (microdochectomy).

A galactocoele is a cystic swelling caused by the retention of milk. It occurs most commonly in the lactating breast in both breast feeding and non-breast feeding mothers. Prolactinomas are tumours of the pituitary gland which may present with galactorrhoea in both men and women.

29. THYROID DISEASE (1)

A – Anaplastic carcinoma
Anaplastic carcinoma is a rare subtype of thyroid cancer (3%) but its incidence increases with age. It is an aggressive carcinoma which often presents with a short history of a lump in the neck with local invasion causing compression of surrounding structures leading to dysphagia, stridor and hoarseness (recurrent laryngeal nerve involvement). Prognosis is poor, with most patients dying within a few months of diagnosis. Treatment is largely palliative and aimed at reducing compressive symptoms. Another rare tumour of the thyroid affecting the older population is lymphoma, which is usually of the non-Hodgkin's type.

The majority (70%) of thyroid tumours are *papillary adenocarcinomas.* Twenty percent are *follicular carcinomas.* Both of these tumours occur most commonly in adolescents and young adults, who present with a discrete thyroid nodule. Papillary tumours may be multifocal and they spread to lymph nodes. Follicular tumours occur as a single encapsulated lesion, and they spread via blood to the lungs and bone. Treatment is by total thyroidectomy (except for tumours <1 cm which require a thyroid lobectomy). Papillary and follicular carcinomas may be TSH-dependent (i.e. the presence of TSH stimulates their growth). For this reason, after thyroid surgery, patients take life-long levothyroxine in order to suppress endogenous TSH secretion and reduce the risk of recurrence.

30. ABDOMINAL PAIN (2)

A – Amylase
This man presents with features highly suggestive of acute pancreatitis. A markedly raised serum amylase (a digestive enzyme produced by the pancreas) would help confirm this diagnosis quickly. The aetiology of acute pancreatitis may be remembered by the mnemonic GET SMASHED:

Gallstones
Ethanol
Trauma
Steroids
Mumps
Autoimmune
Scorpion venom (*Tityus trinitatis* scorpion of Trinidad and Tobago)
Hyperlipidaemia, Hypercalcaemia, Hypothyroidism
Embolism, ERCP
Drugs (azathioprine, steroids, thiazide diuretics and the contraceptive pill)

Pregnancy and pancreatic carcinoma are also causes.

The pathophysiology of acute pancreatitis is as follows: duodeno-pancreatic reflux causes duodenal fluid to enter the pancreas and activate the enzymes within it. This results in autodigestion of the pancreas by trypsin, fat necrosis by lipases and a significant rise in blood amylase. Acute pancreatitis presents with an acute-onset epigastric pain that is *severe* and constant. It characteristically radiates through to the back and is relieved by sitting forward. Patients may also have nausea and vomiting, fever and features of shock. There may be associated inflammatory exudation and peritonitis, presenting with a distended abdomen and absent bowel sounds. The swollen pancreas can block the distal common bile duct, resulting in jaundice. Inflammatory exudates may collect between the stomach and pancreas, resulting in a pancreatic pseudocyst. This classically presents at day 10 of the disease. Extravasation of blood-stained exudates into the retroperitoneum results in a bluish discolouration of the skin. These can be seen as Cullen sign (periumbilical bruising) and Grey Turner sign (flank bruising). These are rarely seen in clinical practice and are not specific to pancreatitis (other causes include blunt abdominal trauma and retroperitoneal haemorrhage). Other useful investigations include an abdominal X-ray which may show a single 'sentinel' loop of air-filled bowel next to the pancreas due to localized ileus, and a CT scan which confirms the diagnosis. Management includes opioid analgesia, intravenous fluids and a proton pump inhibitor.

Antibiotics are not indicated unless disease is severe.

Thomas Stephen Cullen, Canadian gynaecologist (1868–1953).

George Grey Turner, English surgeon (1877–1951).

31. INVESTIGATING ENDOCRINE DISEASE (1)

B – 24-hour urinary vanillylmandelic acid

This woman presents with attacks of anxiety, sweating and palpitations. Along with facial flushing and headaches these are classic presenting features of phaeochromocytomas.

Phaeochromocytomas are tumours of the adrenal medulla (the central part of the adrenal gland). They arise from chromaffin cells and secrete large amounts of catecholamines. Breakdown products of catecholamines include vanillylmandelic acid (VMA), which is excreted in the kidney. Therefore the suspicion of phaeochromocytoma can be strengthened by finding an increased concentration of urinary VMA over a 24-hour period. An abdominal CT will help localize the tumour.

Phaeochromocytomas are associated with a 'ten-percent rule': 10% are malignant, 10% are extra-adrenal, 10% are familial and 10% are bilateral. Familial phaeochromocytomas can be associated with three main conditions: neurofibromatosis, multiple endocrine neoplasia and von Hippel–Lindau syndrome (which is characterized by phaeochromocytomas, retinal haemangioblastomas, clear-cell renal carcinomas and pancreatic neuroendocrine tumours). The treatment of phaeochromocytomas is by surgical excision but, prior to this, alpha-blockers need to be given for

6 weeks to inhibit the effects of a sudden surge of catecholamines that may occur intra-operatively. Life expectancy should be normal if treatment is successful.

Phaeochromocytoma, from Greek *phaios* = dusky brown + *chroma* = colour. This refers to the staining that occurs when these tumours are treated with chromium salts.

32. MANAGING COMMON FRACTURES (1)

D – Intravenous antibiotics and debridement of tissue

An open fracture is an orthopaedic emergency, as fracture communication with the outside environment is a risk for the development of infection both within the soft tissues and bone. As this patient is otherwise stable the first step would be to start broad spectrum antibiotics and debride any large foreign body and necrotic tissue. A tetanus booster is also required. Fixation of the fracture is secondary to wound management in this case. The patient should be prepared to go to theatre as soon as is possible (ideally within 6 hours) for further debridement, washout and fracture stabilization, as the likelihood of infection increases with time.

33. SKIN LESIONS (1)

B – Discoid lupus

Discoid lupus erythematosus (DLE) is a chronic inflammatory condition with an autoimmune aetiology which results in cutaneous manifestations only (unlike systemic lupus erythematosus). In 5% of cases, DLE progresses to the systemic form. Features of discoid lupus are the appearance of well-demarcated erythematous plaque-like lesions most commonly on the cheeks and other sun-exposed areas. Lesions on the scalp destroy hair follicles resulting in alopecia. The palms and soles may also be affected. Symptoms are often exacerbated by sunlight. The plaques heal with significant scarring and can leave areas of depigmentation. Like most autoimmune conditions, discoid lupus is more common in women. Discoid lupus is slightly more common in African-Americans. Presentation is usually in the third to fifth decades. DLE is a relapsing and remitting condition and is treated with topical corticosteroids and hydroxychloroquine. Exposure to UV light must be avoided.

Rosacea is a chronic skin condition that usually affects the face, causing a flushed appearance, but may also affect the neck and upper chest. There is erythema of the skin with papules and pustules. There may be associated conjunctivitis. Unlike DLE, it is most common in the Caucasian population. *Acne vulgaris* is a common condition that affects most people at some point in their lives, commonly during puberty. It is caused by inflammation of the sebaceous glands surrounding hair follicles resulting in the formation of pustules and comedones. There is increased sebum production in response to circulating androgens and the presence of the bacterium *Propionibacterium acnes*. Acne vulgaris can be chronic and cause significant psychological disability. Combination treatment is often required and includes topical and systemic antibacterials, retinoids and hormonal therapies.

34. SHOULDER DISORDERS (1)

D – Posterior dislocation of the shoulder

The shoulder is the most common site affected by dislocations; this is due to its relative instability which allows for its varied range of movements. Posterior dislocation is uncommon, accounting for around 2% of cases. It is most commonly seen in cases of epileptic seizures, electric shocks and following a direct blow to the front of the shoulder. The arm will be held internally rotated and adducted, and there is resistance to external rotation. The humeral head will be palpable posteriorly below the acromion. The AP view on X-ray will show an abnormally rounded appearance of the humeral head (the 'light bulb sign') but diagnosis of dislocation is confirmed on the lateral view. Closed reduction is possible under appropriate sedation.

Anterior dislocation (98%) is usually caused by a fall onto the outstretched arm or the shoulder itself. The arm will be held in external rotation and abduction. The humeral head is felt anteriorly beneath the clavicle. Diagnosis is best made on AP view. There is associated neurovascular injury in 5%, so it is important also to examine the integrity of the axillary nerve (sensation over the upper lateral aspect of the arm – the regimental badge area). Various methods of closed reduction may be used (e.g. Kocher manoeuvre). *Inferior dislocation,* known as 'luxatio erecta', is a very rare dislocation caused by hyperabduction injuries. The patient presents with the arm in full abduction with the elbow fully flexed ('hand behind the head'). These dislocations are frequently associated with fractures and there is a higher incidence of neurovascular injury than with anterior dislocations.

Acromioclavicular dislocations are usually caused by a direct fall onto the shoulder and may be associated with a fractured clavicle. A step may be felt at the point of separation, which is confirmed on AP X-ray. Treatment may be conservative with immobilization using a sling or 'strapping', or operative in which a screw is used to bring the clavicle and coracoid process together. *Sternoclavicular dislocations* are rare. The majority are anterior (90%) and caused by a direct blow to the shoulder. The medial head of the clavicle may be easily palpated with such dislocations. Sternoclavicular dislocations are difficult to see on the standard AP and lateral views, and may require 'serendipity views', which are focused on the sternoclavicular joints. Treatment is usually conservative in anterior sternoclavicular dislocations (sling), but posterior dislocations must be promptly reduced.

35. MANAGING VENOUS DISEASE (1)

A – Debridement and intravenous antibiotics

Varicose veins are a result of incompetent valves between the deep and superficial venous systems, leading to venous hypertension, insufficiency and ulceration. Incompetence occurs in around one in ten of the population, with approximately 0.2% developing venous ulcers (95% being around the malleoli 'gaiter area'). Other skin changes associated with incompetence are venous eczema and lipodermatosclerosis. The mainstay of treatment of venous ulcers is graded compression bandaging with high pressure at the ankle tapering at the knee. There is a recurrence rate of ulcers of 20% and definitive cure can only be achieved by stripping incompetent veins. In this case, the patient has an infected ulcer with systemic upset and therefore requires intravenous antibiotics. Debridement of non-viable tissue aids healing of the ulcer. Sclerotherapy is used for treatment of spider veins and uncomplicated varicose veins.

36. CUTANEOUS MALIGNANCIES (1)

A – Acral lentiginous melanoma

Malignant melanomas are malignant tumours of melanocytes. Although they are one of the rarer forms of skin cancer they have a high mortality. Acral lentiginous melanoma is one of the rarer subtypes of malignant melanoma (5%) but accounts for at least half of all melanoma in those with dark skin (Asians, Afro-Caribbeans). It typically presents from the seventh decade and is found in hairless areas – palms, soles of feet, under the nails and in the buccal mucosa. The lesions may initially be mistaken for bruises and those under the nail for 'benign' nail streaks. As a result, presentation of this subtype of melanoma is often late.

The most common form of malignant melanoma is the *superficial spreading* type which usually occurs in a pre-existing mole but may also occur *de novo*. It is most common in Caucasian women and occurs on sun-exposed areas such as the legs, neck and trunk. It is initially a flat irregular lesion which may be pigmented to varying degrees. Itching and bleeding occur with spread. Superficial spreading malignant melanoma is the leading cause of death from cancer in young adults. *Nodular melanomas* arise *de novo* and present as a nodular pigmented lesion. They grow rapidly, extending deeper into the tissue than can be seen on the surface. Nodular melanomas are the most aggressive subtype of malignant melanomas. *Lentigo maligna melanomas* develop within an area of pigmented sun-damaged skin and progress over a period of years into a malignant lesion. The development of nodules or irregular borders within or around a pre-existing area of pigmentation suggests lentigo melanoma. *Amelanocytic melanomas* are melanomas which are unpigmented. As they are subtle in appearance they are not as easily noticed and hence have a poorer prognosis.

Malignant melanomas are diagnosed on skin biopsy and staged according to their thickness (Breslow classification) and depth of invasion into the skin layers (Clark's classification).

Mohs micrographic surgery (MMS) is often used by dermatologists to excise skin lesions. Here one undertakes intra-operative pathological tissue assessment to ensure clear resection margins.

Frederic Edward Mohs, American physician and general surgeon (1910–2002).

37. NECK LUMPS (1)

A – Branchial cyst

Branchial cysts arise from the embryonic remnants of the second branchial cleft, secondary to cystic degeneration of lymphoid tissue. They are commoner in males on the left side. A branchial cyst is a smooth, non-tender, fluctuant swelling in the anterior triangle, anterior to the border of the sternocleidomastoid muscle at the junction of its upper and middle thirds. The cyst may enlarge following an upper respiratory tract infection. Unlike cystic hygromas, they do not transilluminate. Branchial cysts may become enlarged and tender with upper respiratory tract infections. Diagnosis is by aspiration which demonstrates a creamy fluid containing cholesterol crystals. Treatment is by excision.

Ischaemic contracture of the sternocleidomastoid muscle can occur due to birth trauma and often presents after a few weeks of life with tilting of the head (torticollis) and a painless fibrous mass in the sternocleidomastoid muscle (*sternocleidomastoid tumour*). Treatment is by passive stretching of the muscle, and the swelling eventually disappears by the sixth month of life.

A *cervical rib* is a congenital overdevelopment of the transverse process of the C7 vertebra. This so-called 'rib' can interfere with the lower roots of the brachial plexus (T1), the sympathetic nerves and the subclavian artery. If the T1 root of the brachial plexus is affected, there is pain and paraesthesia in the T1 distribution (medial aspect of the arm) and wasting of the small muscles of the hand (also supplied by T1). Disturbance of the sympathetic nerves results in a Horner syndrome (ipsilateral miosis, ptosis, enophthalmos and anhidrosis). If the subclavian artery is pinched by the cervical rib, there will be a stenosis and reduced blood flow to the arm. This becomes apparent on exertion because when the arm needs more blood it will 'steal' it from the vertebral artery (which should supply the brain). Therefore if the affected arm is exerted a loss of consciousness may result. This phenomenon is known as the 'subclavian steal syndrome'. Diagnosis of a cervical rib is by X-ray of the cervical spine. Treatment is by excision.

Torticollis, from Latin *torti* = twist + *collis* = neck.

Johann Friedrich Horner, Swedish ophthalmologist (1831–1886).

38. COMPLICATIONS OF NASAL FRACTURE

E – Septal haematoma

The formation of a septal haematoma is a rare but recognized complication of nasal fractures, resulting from the collection of blood between the perichondrium and the nasal cartilage. The haematoma disrupts the blood supply to the cartilage which, together with pressure effect, results in necrosis and deformity. The haematoma may also become infected resulting in an abscess. Following a nasal injury, it is important to assess for an intranasal/septal haematoma which is detected as a 'cherry red' mass. If it is present, the patient must be referred for urgent aspiration or drainage together with prophylactic antibiotics. Fracture of both the cribriform plate and orbital wall ('blowout fractures') can occur with direct nasal trauma. Cribriform fractures can cause CSF to leak from the nose (CSF rhinorrhoea). If this is present, antibiotics must be commenced and a neurosurgical opinion sought due to the risk of developing meningitis. If there is a suspicion of a basal skull/cribriform plate fracture in a trauma scenario, under no circumstances should an NG tube be passed.

Orbital fractures can present with infra-orbital and upper lip/gum numbness (caused by damage to the infraorbital nerve) and diplopia (caused by herniation of the ocular muscle through the fracture or compression by a surrounding haematoma). Facial X-rays are not particularly sensitive for isolated nasal fractures but must be obtained if there is any suspicion of fractures of other facial bones. CT may also be required, especially if there is suspicion of a cribriform fracture. Uncomplicated fractures of the nose can be reduced and a septoplasty performed once swelling has settled (usually after a week).

39. MANAGING TESTICULAR PAIN (1)

C – Contact the urologist on call and prepare for theatre

This patient has presented with an acutely painful testicle and torsion of the testis must be confirmed or excluded by exploration. A Doppler ultrasound can confirm the diagnosis but will delay definitive treatment and therefore, in any potential case of torsion, time must not be wasted in trying to obtain a scan. The testis will remain viable if explored and fixed within 6 hours but, if delayed to 12 hours, the viability rate is around one in five. Testicular torsion is a urological emergency with an incidence of 1/4000 in males under the age of 25, and a peak incidence between the ages of 12 and 18 years. Other causes of an acutely painful scrotum include torsion of the testicular appendage (hydatid of Morgagni), acute epididymitis and strangulated inguinal hernias.

Torsions can only be definitively diagnosed or excluded upon operative scrotal exploration. Clinical features to be gleaned from history and examination include: testicular tenderness (ischaemic testes are very tender unless they are dead); the lie and height of the testis in the scrotum (a high testis with a transverse lie in relation to the other testis may well be torted – feel for a 'knot' in the cord); any scrotal erythema or discolouration; the presence or absence of the cremasteric reflex or swelling of the scrotum (the cremasteric reflex is often attenuated in torsion and of the available clinical signs this is the most sensitive, but it is still not definitive).

40. CHEST TRAUMA (1)

B – Insert a wide-bore cannula into the second intercostal space

This patient has a tension pneumothorax. Air entering the pleural cavity during inspiration cannot escape during expiration due to the pleura acting as a one-way valve. Tension pneumothorax is an emergency, as the buildup of air compresses the lung, preventing expansion. Symptoms include breathlessness and chest pain, and on examination there is tachypnoea, hypotension, reduced expansion and air entry on the affected side of the chest, hyperresonance to percussion and deviation of the trachea and apex to the opposite side. If not decompressed urgently, cardiorespiratory collapse and death can ensue within minutes. Decompression is by insertion of a large bore cannula into the second intercostal space in the mid-clavicular line of the affected side. A gush of air will be heard as the pressure is released. A formal chest drain can then be inserted (5th intercostal space of the mid-axillary line). Do not waste time obtaining a chest X-ray if the diagnosis is suspected. Treatment should be based on clinical findings. A pericardiocentesis is performed in the management of cardiac tamponade.

41. EYE DISEASE (1)

D – Topical pilocarpine

This patient has presented with acute closed angle glaucoma which, if not urgently treated, can result in blindness within 24 hours. It is caused by a blockage in the drainage of aqueous humour from the anterior chamber of the eye via the canal of Schlemm, resulting in an increase in the intraocular pressure. This occurs acutely when the pupil dilates and the iris comes into contact with the trabecular meshwork which is found at the entrance to the canal of Schlemm, such as when watching television in the dark. Acute glaucoma is most common after middle age and may also occur as a chronic or subacute condition, where it is associated with a shallow anterior chamber, long sightedness and thickening of the lens. The immediate treatment of acute closed angle glaucoma is with pilocarpine eye drops. Pilocarpine is a selective muscarinic receptor agonist which causes miosis (papillary constriction), opening up the entrance to the canal of Schlemm. Intraocular pressure may also be decreased by the use of intravenous acetazolamide, which reduces the production of aqueous humour. Acute closed angle glaucoma warrants an urgent ophthalmological referral. Once the acute attack is controlled, an iridectomy is performed to allow free circulation of aqueous humour and prevent further attacks.

Friedrich Schlemm, German anatomist (1795–1858).

42. PAEDIATRIC ORTHOPAEDICS (1)

B – Irritable hip

Transient synovitis (irritable hip) is the most common cause of acute hip pain in pre-pubescent children (usually 6 months to 6 years) and often follows a viral infection. Features include sudden onset hip pain that radiates to the knee, a slight limp and a reduced range of movement, especially external rotation. There is no pain at rest and minimal systemic symptoms. Investigations, such as full blood count, acute phase proteins, joint X-ray and blood cultures, are negative. Ultrasound investigation may demonstrate a small effusion. Management is with analgesia, bed rest and skin traction. Irritable hip usually resolves in 7–10 days. In a septic arthritis there will be fever and raised inflammatory markers.

43. INVESTIGATING DYSPHAGIA (1)

D – Tensilon test

This patient presents with signs and symptoms of myasthenia gravis. Myasthenia gravis is an autoimmune condition characterized by muscle weakness and fatigability. It is caused by autoantibodies to acetylcholine receptors at the postsynaptic neuromuscular junction, thereby reducing the stimulative effect of acetylcholine. The most common muscles to be affected are those of the eyes and face, although the condition may progress to affect respiratory muscle function – a myasthenic crisis. (This is a medical emergency which requires artificial ventilation.) The gold standard investigation for diagnosing myasthenia gravis is the Tensilon test. Tensilon is the trade name for edrophonium bromide, a short-acting anti-cholinesterase, which, when administered intravenously, transiently improves muscle weakness by allowing the prolonged action of acetylcholine. The effects are best seen after asking the patient to perform repetitive movements to cause muscle fatigue.

Creatine kinase is an enzyme expressed by various muscular tissues, including smooth muscle. Levels are detected on blood testing and a higher than normal level is associated with muscular damage, e.g. following rhabdomyolysis and myocardial infarction. Troponin is an enzyme that is only found in skeletal and cardiac muscle. It is detected easily on blood testing and is commonly used to diagnose myocardial infarction, as it is more specific than creatine kinase. Electromyography is used to detect and record the action potential generated by muscles in both their contracted and relaxed state. It can be used in the diagnosis of both muscular and nerve conditions, e.g. carpal tunnel syndrome and Duchenne muscular dystrophy. Muscle biopsy allows histological examination of tissue and may be used to identify and differentiate between various myopathies. The latter two investigations often complement each other.

44. INVESTIGATING UROLOGICAL DISEASE (1)

E – Urgent referral for transrectal ultrasound and prostate biopsy

This patient has presented with symptoms of bladder outflow obstruction, the most common cause in this age group being prostatic hypertrophy. Most cases of prostatic hypertrophy are benign and can be treated medically or surgically if symptoms are severe and persistent. In this case, the patient's prostate specific antigen (PSA) is markedly elevated (normal values in this age group being 5 or below) and he would therefore need further investigation with prostate biopsy to exclude malignancy. Other causes of a raised PSA include urinary tract infection. Digital rectal examination and ejaculation within the last 48 hours can also marginally raise PSA.

45. ABDOMINAL PAIN (3)

C – Diverticulitis

A diverticulum is an outpouching of a hollow structure. Colonic diverticula are examples of false diverticula – the walls are made up only of the inner mucosal layer of the bowel. A true diverticulum involves all the layers of the wall from which it arises, e.g. Meckel diverticulum. Diverticulosis describes the presence of colonic diverticula. Diverticular disease is a term used if complications arise from diverticulosis. Finally, diverticulitis specifically describes inflammation of the diverticula.

Colonic diverticula are most commonly found in the sigmoid and the descending colon. They are unusual in the under-40s, but 30% of the elderly populations of developed countries are found to have diverticulosis at autopsy. The pathogenesis of diverticulosis is as follows: there is hypertrophy of the muscle of the sigmoid colon, resulting in high intraluminal pressures. This leads to herniation of the mucosa at potential sites of weakness in the bowel wall, which correspond to points of entry of blood vessels. The underlying aetiology of the initial large bowel hypertrophy is unknown, but it may be directly due to a diet that is chronically low in fibre. Complications of diverticulosis include diverticulitis, lower gastrointestinal haemorrhage from erosion of a blood vessel within a diverticulum, and obstruction from chronic diverticular infection and fibrosis. The diagnosis of diverticulosis is made by flexible sigmoidoscopy. Barium enema shows the diverticular outpouchings with a signet ring appearance due to filling defects produced by pellets of faeces within the diverticula. In the acute phase of suspected diverticulitis, CT is the best investigation. Treatment of diverticulitis is largely conservative; patients are nil by mouth with the administration of intravenous fluids and antibiotics until symptoms improve. Complications of diverticulitis include the formation of abscesses (which may perforate leading to peritonitis), fistulae and strictures.

Constipation, which predisposes to diverticulosis, is a common cause of lower abdominal pain; however it is not associated with any inflammatory response. Another complication of chronic constipation is a sigmoid volvulus, where the loop of chronically distended, atonic bowel twists around its mesenteric axis. *Irritable bowel syndrome* is caused by a functional abnormality of the bowel which is most common in young women. Typical symptoms include bouts of colicky pain, bloating and an abnormal bowel habit, and tend to occur intermittently. The passage of blood in the stools is *never* due to irritable bowel syndrome. The cause is unknown but there are associations with stress and poor diet. Investigations are performed not to diagnose irritable bowel syndrome, but to exclude other pathology. Treatment is largely symptomatic.

46. BONE TUMOURS (1)

E – Osteosarcoma

Osteosarcomas are the second most common primary bone tumours after multiple myeloma. Osteosarcomas occur most often in young adults, in which case they may be associated with a history of retinoblastoma, and in older people with Paget disease. Osteosarcoma is twice as common in males. Osteosarcomas present with a warm, painful swelling, usually around the knee (50%). The pain tends to be worse at night. X-ray features are characteristic, showing cortical destruction, periosteal elevation (Codman's triangle) and calcification within the tumour but outside of the bone (sunray spicules). Diagnosis is confirmed by biopsy, and treatment is by neoadjuvant chemotherapy with radical surgery. Osteosarcomas are *very* malignant tumours and blood-borne metastases develop early and spread to the lungs (around 30% by time of diagnosis).

47. HAEMATURIA

D – Transitional cell carcinoma

Renal calculi, cystitis and urethral injury generally cause painful haematuria, and diverticulitis is a cause of rectal bleeding. Transitional cell carcinomas (TCC) are the most common form of bladder cancer in Europe, accounting for more than 90% of all bladder cancers. Other types of bladder cancer include squamous cell carcinoma, which is more common in the developing world secondary to infection with *Schistosoma haematobium,* and adenocarcinomas. Bladder TCC occurs most commonly in the sixties, with a male to female ratio of 3:1. There is a strong association with smoking and exposure to aromatic amines in dyes. Bladder TCC usually presents with frank painless haematuria, though rarely it presents with irritative symptoms, obstruction and symptoms of metastasis such as bony pain. Up to 10% of patients may present with only microscopic haematuria. Diagnosis is made on histology of biopsy of suspicious lesions found on cystoscopy. The majority of TCCs are superficial on presentation (70%). Treatment depends on the staging of the cancer and can involve transurethral resection of the bladder tumour, intravesical BCG or chemotherapy, and radical cystectomy. There is a high recurrence rate of superficial TCC (up to 70%), so close follow-up with repeat cystoscopies is warranted.

48. THE SWOLLEN LIMB (1)

E – Milroy disease

Lymphoedema is an accumulation of tissue fluid within the extracellular compartment due to a failure in the lymphatic system. Most cases (80%) occur in the lower limbs. Lymphoedema should be contrasted with oedema, which is an accumulation of tissue fluid in the absence of a lymphatic abnormality.

Primary lymphoedema is commoner in females and in those with a family history. It is classified according to the age of onset: congenital (Milroy disease – an inherited autosomal dominant congenital lymphoedema, caused by a failure of lymph vessels to develop in utero); lymphoedema praecox (presents under 35 years); and lymphoedema tarda (presents over 35 years). Isotope lymphography, where a radioactive tracer is injected subcutaneously into the foot and its progress monitored, can be performed. A delayed transit time confirms the diagnosis. Management options for primary lymphoedema include compression, elevation, aggressive antibiotic therapy for infections and debulking surgery (indicated when conservative treatment has failed).

William Forsyth Milroy, American physician (1855–1942).

49. PAEDIATRIC SURGICAL MANAGEMENT (1)

D – Incision and drainage with intravenous antibiotics

This boy has presented with the symptoms and signs of a psoas abscess. A psoas abscess may be primary (and commonly caused by *Staphylococcus aureus*) or secondary to spread of infection from structures adjacent to the muscle, e.g. from a tuberculous paraspinal abscess (Pott's disease). Presenting features are often non-specific and include flank, abdominal, hip and thigh pain associated with a fever and limp. Any action which causes the flexion or contraction of the psoas muscle results in pain. Note that on the right side this may also be a sign of acute appendicitis. Diagnosis may be confirmed on CT or MRI and treatment is with appropriate antimicrobial therapy along with incision and drainage of the abscess.

50. UPPER LIMB PAIN

A – Median nerve

This patient has presented with the symptoms and signs of carpal tunnel syndrome, which results from compression of the median nerve in the carpal tunnel of the wrist. Being the only soft tissue structure in this region, it is susceptible to compression. The median nerve supplies sensation to the palm of the hand and the radial three and a half fingers. Motor supply of the nerve is to the lateral two lumbricals, opponens pollicis, abductor pollicis brevis and flexor pollicis brevis ('LOAF'). Carpal tunnel commonly presents in the forties and is more common in women. Most cases are idiopathic but it can occur in pregnancy, hypothyroidism, rheumatoid arthritis, acromegaly and following Colles fracture. The symptoms of carpal tunnel can be precipitated by sudden forced palmar flexion of the wrist (Phalen test) or by tapping *over* the site of the median nerve at the wrist (Tinel test). Treatment may initially include rest, analgesia and splinting; however, if symptoms do not resolve, decompression surgery is indicated.

Jules Tinel, French neurologist (1879–1952).

George Phalen, American orthopaedic surgeon (1911–1998).

Practice Paper 2: Questions

1. ABDOMINAL INCISIONS (1)

A 45-year-old woman has been diagnosed with gallstones. She opts to have an open cholecystectomy.

Which of the following surgical incisions would be most appropriate?

A. Gridiron
B. Lanz
C. Right Kocher's
D. Right paramedian
E. Rooftop

2. SHOCK (2)

A 56-year-old woman is brought into the resuscitation room. Three days ago she suffered an insect bite to the abdomen which has now spread, causing redness across the whole of her abdomen. On examination, she is confused, with a temperature of 38.3°C, heart rate 106/min and blood pressure 100/56 mmHg.

Which of the following is specific to the treatment of this type of shock?

A. Antibiotics
B. Antihistamines
C. Atropine
D. Fluids
E. Inotropes

3. UPPER GI BLEED (2)

A 21-year-old girl has been out drinking with her friends. She is escorted into hospital by the paramedics after vomiting up a large amount of fresh blood. She is normally fit and well.

Which of the following is the most likely cause?

A. Boerhaave syndrome
B. Epistaxis
C. Haemoptysis
D. Mallory–Weiss tear
E. Oesophageal varices

4. BONE TUMOURS (2)

A 15-year-old boy attends the emergency department with a 2-week history of pain in the left lower leg and fever. On examination, there is a tender, irregular swelling of the tibia. X-ray of the leg shows a lytic lesion with a laminated periosteal reaction.

What is the most likely diagnosis?

A. Chondrosarcoma
B. Enchondroma
C. Ewing sarcoma
D. Osteoid osteoma
E. Osteosarcoma

5. BILIARY TRACT DISEASE (2)

A 72-year-old woman presents to the emergency department with a 5-hour history of abdominal pain, bloating and vomiting. On examination, the abdomen is distended and auscultation reveals intermittent high-pitched sounds. An abdominal X-ray shows air in the biliary tree.

What is the most likely diagnosis?

A. Emphysematous cholecystitis
B. Gallstone ileus
C. Paralytic ileus
D. Perforated gallbladder
E. Pyogenic cholecystitis

6. CUTANEOUS MALIGNANCIES (2)

A 52-year-old man presents to the GP complaining of an enlarging lump on his face. On examination, he has a 1 cm pigmented, raised lesion on his left cheek that has a shiny rolled edge.

What is the most likely diagnosis?

A. Basal cell carcinoma
B. Bowen disease
C. Keratoacanthoma
D. Seborrhoeic keratosis
E. Squamous cell carcinoma

7. MANAGING ANORECTAL DISEASE (2)

A 43-year-old woman presents with bright red fresh rectal bleeding and intermittent rectal discomfort. She has recently noticed a mass in her rectum. On examination, a non-tender lump is seen emerging from the rectum. It cannot be reduced.

Which of the following would be the most appropriate treatment?

A. Anal dilatation
B. Banding

C. Haemorrhoidectomy
D. Injection sclerotherapy
E. No intervention required

8. INVESTIGATING ENDOCRINE DISEASE (2)

A 42-year-old woman presents to the emergency department with difficulty breathing and facial flushing which began soon after having a few drinks at the pub. She tells you that she has had a few of these episodes recently, always after having an alcoholic drink. Examination is unremarkable. Her observations include: heart rate 82/min and blood pressure 122/86 mmHg.

Which investigation will most likely confirm the underlying diagnosis?

A. 17-hydroxyprogesterone levels
B. 24-hour urinary vanillylmandelic acid
C. 24-hour urinary 5-hydroxyindole acetic acid
D. Serum calcitonin
E. Short synacthen test

9. HERNIAS (2)

A 62-year-old man presents to the GP with a lump in the left groin which has been present for over 2 months. On examination, the lump is above the inguinal ligament. It is reducible and has a cough impulse, but does not extend into the scrotum.

Which of the following is the most likely diagnosis?

A. Direct inguinal hernia
B. Femoral hernia
C. Gluteal hernia
D. Indirect inguinal hernia
E. Obturator hernia

10. GROIN LUMPS (2)

A 44-year-old man presents to the GP having noticed a painless swelling in the right side of the scrotum. On examination, the scrotum is swollen and non-tender. The swelling transilluminates and the testis itself is not palpable.

What is the most likely diagnosis?

A. Epididymo-orchitis
B. Hydrocele
C. Inguinal hernia
D. Testicular torsion
E. Varicocele

11. BREAST DISEASE (2)

A 27-year-old woman presents to the GP with a single lump in the left breast that has been present for 6 months. On examination, there is a 3 cm smooth lump in the upper outer quadrant of the breast that is mobile and not attached to the overlying skin.

What is the most likely diagnosis?

A. Breast abscess
B. Breast cyst
C. Fibroadenoma
D. Gynaecomastia
E. Phyllodes tumour

12. PAEDIATRIC SURGICAL MANAGEMENT (2)

A 6-month-old boy is brought into the emergency department by his parents. He appears to have been having paroxysms of intense pain since that morning, described by his parents as episodes of crying and drawing of his legs up to the abdomen. This evening he has passed some mucus-like blood from the back passage. His temperature is 36.8°C.

Which of the following would be the best treatment option in the first instance?

A. Barium enema
B. Continued observation
C. Intravenous antibiotics
D. Laparotomy
E. Scrotal exploration

13. ARTERIAL BLOOD GASES (2)

A 67-year-old woman presents to the emergency department with a 1-month history of malaise, weight loss, worsening cough and haemoptysis. You notice her saturations are 92% on air and perform a blood gas test with the following results: pH 7.37, pO_2 6.7, pCO_2 7.4, bicarbonate 35, saturations 91.7%.

Reference ranges: pO_2 >11.0 kPa, pCO_2 4.6–6.0 kPa, bicarbonate 22–28 mmol/L, pH 7.35–7.45.

What blood gas picture does this represent?

A. Fully compensated metabolic acidosis
B. Fully compensated metabolic alkalosis
C. Fully compensated respiratory acidosis
D. Type I respiratory failure
E. Venous sample

14. JAUNDICE (2)

A 40-year-old woman presents to the emergency department with a 4-hour history of right upper abdominal pain and fever. She tells you that she has previously been investigated for abdominal pain and was found to have gall-stones. She says that she has never felt this unwell with the pain before. On examination, she is markedly jaundiced with a temperature of 39°C and pulse rate of 130/min. There is localized peritonism in the right upper abdomen.

Which of the following complications of gallstones has this patient presented with?

A. Acute cholecystitis
B. Ascending cholangitis
C. Biliary colic
D. Carcinoma of the gallbladder
E. Gallstone ileus

15. PREOPERATIVE MORBIDITY (2)

A 56-year-old man presents to the pre-assessment clinic prior to an elective knee operation. He tells you he smokes 20 cigarettes a day and suffers from occasional angina.

Which of the following best describes his preoperative morbidity?

A. ASA grade I
B. ASA grade II
C. ASA grade III
D. ASA grade IV
E. ASA grade V

16. THYROID DISEASE (2)

A 41-year-old woman presents to the GP with a 1-week history of feeling tired, muscle aches, neck pain and restlessness. On examination, she has a smooth enlarged thyroid. Her heart rate is 120/min and blood pressure 128/88 mmHg, with a temperature of 37.3°C.

What is the most likely diagnosis?

A. De Quervain thyroiditis
B. Hashimoto thyroiditis
C. Pharyngitis
D. Riedel thyroiditis
E. Thyroglossal cyst

17. ABDOMINAL PAIN (4)

A 33-year-old man presents with a 2-hour history of upper abdominal pain that radiates to his back and shoulders. On examination, he is sweaty and his abdomen is rigid. His observations include heart rate 106/min and blood pressure 98/58 mmHg.

Which of the following is the most likely cause of his symptoms?

A. Epigastric hernia incarceration
B. Gastric carcinoma

C. Gastritis
D. Hiatus hernia
E. Perforated peptic ulcer

18. FLUID THERAPY (1)

A 43-year-old man is brought into the resuscitation room having been involved in a house fire. On arrival you estimate him to have 20% burns. The man is around 80 kg in weight.

How much fluid should the patient have over the next 12 hours?

A. 300 mL
B. 600 mL
C. 1200 mL
D. 2400 mL
E. 3000 mL

19. ENDOCRINE DISEASE (2)

A 17-year-old boy is referred to the endocrinology clinic with a 1-month history of paroxysmal sweating, anxiety and palpitations. He has had a thyroid tumour in the past which was successfully resected. On examination, you notice that he is tall and thin with long fingers.

What is the most likely diagnosis?

A. Carcinoid syndrome
B. Multiple endocrine neoplasia type I
C. Multiple endocrine neoplasia type IIa
D. Multiple endocrine neoplasia type IIb
E. Nelson syndrome

20. MANAGING ABDOMINAL PAIN (2)

A 54-year-old woman has been having episodes of epigastric pain associated with food. She is referred for an endoscopy which shows gastric ulceration. A rapid urease test performed on a biopsy sample is positive.

Which of the following would you use to treat this patient?

A. Augmentin and metronidazole
B. Omeprazole, clarithromycin and metronidazole
C. Omeprazole, prednisolone and augmentin
D. Omeprazole and ibuprofen
E. Ranitidine

21. SKIN LESIONS (2)

A 7-month-old boy is taken by his parents to the GP with a red lesion on his scalp which has been enlarging over the past 2 months. On examination, the lesion is 1 cm in size, raised, bright red and well defined. The boy is otherwise well.

What is the most likely diagnosis?

A. Cavernous haemangioma
B. Deep capillary naevus
C. Dercum disease
D. Pyogenic granuloma
E. Superficial capillary naevus

22. NECK LUMPS (2)

A 12-month-old girl is brought to the GP by her mother with a large mass in the right side of her neck which she has noticed for a few months. On examination, the mass is fleshy and compressible, and lies posterior to the right sternocleidomastoid.
What is the most likely diagnosis?

A. Branchial cyst
B. Cystic hygroma
C. Pleomorphic adenoma
D. Sternocleidomastoid tumour
E. Thyroglossal cyst

23. CONDITIONS OF THE NOSE

A 3-year-old boy is brought into the GP practice by his father. The child has had a yellowish discharge from his right nostril for the last 3 days. Examination of the nostril is difficult as the child is distressed, but you see what appears to be a small piece of plastic.
Which of the following would you do?

A. Continue to try to remove the foreign body yourself
B. Give oral antibiotics and see the child in a week
C. Perform cauterization
D. Perform nasal packing
E. Refer to ENT on call to remove foreign body

24. ABDOMINAL PAIN (5)

A 24-year-old woman presents to the emergency department complaining of a 2-day history of lower abdominal pain with associated foul-smelling vaginal discharge. On examination, she is tender and guarding in both the suprapubic region and the right iliac fossa. A urine dipstick shows leukocytes and protein.
What is the most likely diagnosis?

A. Appendicitis
B. Ectopic pregnancy
C. Mittelschmerz
D. Pelvic inflammatory disease
E. Urinary tract infection

25. COMPLICATIONS OF COLLES FRACTURES

A 64-year-old woman who was conservatively treated in plaster for a Colles fracture re-presents to the fracture clinic 2 weeks after plaster removal complaining of a burning pain in the whole hand. On examination, the hand is slightly swollen, red and shiny. There is a reduction in all hand and finger movements.

Which of the following is most likely to be the cause of her symptoms?

A. Carpal tunnel syndrome
B. Compartment syndrome
C. Malunion of the fracture
D. Rupture of the extensor pollicis longus
E. Sudeck atrophy

26. KNEE INJURIES

A 26-year-old man has been referred to the fracture clinic with instability of the left knee. His symptoms followed a football injury in which he heard a 'pop' in his knee while being tackled. He tells you that he attended the emergency department immediately and a large amount of blood was drained from the knee.

On examination which of the following would you expect to find?

A. Positive Lachman test
B. Positive McMurray test
C. Positive Simmonds test
D. Positive patellar apprehension test
E. Valgus instability of the knee joint

27. CHEST TRAUMA (2)

A 32-year-old man is involved in a high speed car accident. On arrival at the resuscitation room he complains of chest pain and is short of breath and tachycardic. He has an area of paradoxical movement of the chest wall.

Which of the following would be the most appropriate management measure?

A. Analgesia and respiratory support
B. Chest drain insertion
C. Needle thoracocentesis
D. Pericardiocentesis
E. Thoracotomy

28. EYE DISEASE (2)

A 47-year-old man presents to the emergency department with a 2-day history of a painful, watery, red left eye. On examination, the cornea is injected and examination under cobalt-blue light after the instillation of fluorescein, reveals a branch-like corneal lesion.

Which of the following is the most likely diagnosis?

A. Anterior uveitis
B. Bacterial conjunctivitis
C. Corneal abrasion
D. Episcleritis
E. Herpes simplex keratitis

29. HEPATOMEGALY (2)

A 62-year-old smoker presents with a 2-week history of worsening shortness of breath, haemoptysis and weight loss. On examination, he appears cachexic and his liver is enlarged with an irregular border.

Which of the following is the most likely cause of his hepatomegaly?

A. Budd-Chiari syndrome
B. Hepatocellular carcinoma
C. Liver cirrhosis
D. Metastatic liver disease
E. Riedel lobe

30. NIPPLE DISCHARGE (2)

A 34-year-old woman presents to the GP with a 3-week history of left nipple discharge. She describes the discharge as thick and greenish. On examination, no mass is palpable within the breast. A beta-hCG urine test is negative.

What is the most likely diagnosis?

A. Breast cancer
B. Duct ectasia
C. Intraductal papilloma
D. Lactating breast
E. Prolactinoma

31. PAEDIATRIC SURGERY (2)

A 1-day-old baby girl is having repeated bile-stained vomiting. Her mother was noted to have polyhydramnios during the pregnancy. An abdominal X-ray reveals gas in the stomach and first part of the duodenum, but nowhere else in the abdomen.

What is the most likely diagnosis?

A. Choledochal cyst
B. Duodenal atresia
C. Oesophageal atresia
D. Pyloric stenosis
E. Renal agenesis

32. INVESTIGATING ABDOMINAL PAIN (2)

A 73-year-old man presents to the emergency department with sudden-onset right-sided back pain radiating to the abdomen. He has a past medical history of hypertension and angina and is known to have gallstones. On examination, he is afebrile, haemodynamically stable and tender in the right side of the abdomen. Blood tests show normal inflammatory markers. Urine dipstick shows a trace of blood.

What investigation would you perform next?

A. CT abdomen
B. Intravenous urogram
C. Laparotomy
D. MRI spine
E. Ultrasound abdomen

33. VASCULAR DISEASE (2)

A 21-year-old man presents to the emergency department with a collapse that was preceded by dizziness and right arm pain. He was sanding a table at home when the event happened. On examination, he has a bony lump palpable in the right side of the neck. Neurological and vascular examinations are otherwise normal.

What is the most likely diagnosis?

A. Cerebrovascular attack
B. Deep venous thrombosis
C. Embolus
D. Subclavian steal syndrome
E. Transient ischaemic attack

34. LOWER LIMB NERVE LESIONS (2)

A 42-year-old woman is taken to theatre after fracturing her left hip in a road traffic collision. Postoperatively, it is noticed that she is unable to flex or extend her left foot. There is no sensation present below the left knee except over the medial aspect of the leg.

Which nerve has most likely been affected?

A. Common peroneal nerve
B. Femoral nerve
C. Sciatic nerve
D. Sural nerve
E. Saphenous nerve

35. INVESTIGATING UROLOGICAL DISEASE (2)

A 33-year-old man comes to see you at the GP surgery complaining of increasing difficulty passing urine with poor flow. He has previously been treated for gonorrhoea on three separate occasions.

Which of the following investigations would be most useful in establishing the cause of his symptoms?

A. Intravenous urogram
B. Ultrasound of the renal tract
C. Urethral swabs
D. Urethrography
E. Urinary flow rates

36. SPINAL CORD LESIONS (2)

A 76-year-old man presents to the emergency department after a fall. He now feels weak in his arms and legs. On examination, he has mild weakness in both arms, and a moderate weakness in the legs. He is unable to feel pain in his legs.

What is the most likely diagnosis?

A. Anterior cord syndrome
B. Brown-Séquard syndrome
C. Central cord syndrome
D. Posterior cord syndrome
E. Syringomyelia

37. TUMOUR MARKERS (2)

A 54-year-old man presents with a recent change in bowel habit associated with a constant desire to defaecate. He has lost two stone in weight over the last month and feels lethargic.

Which of the following tumour markers would be associated with his condition?

A. CA 125
B. CA 15-3
C. CA 19-9
D. CEA
E. PSA

38. MANAGING TESTICULAR PAIN (2)

An 8-year-old boy is brought into the emergency department with a 3-day history of right-sided testicular pain. His mother tells you he was off school a week ago with complaints of feeling unwell and jaw pain on eating. On examination, there is unilateral generalized swelling and tenderness of the right testis.

Which of the following treatment options is most appropriate?

A. Analgesia and bed rest
B. Antibiotics
C. Hydrocelectomy
D. Orchidectomy
E. Reduction and fixation of testis

ANORECTAL DISEASE (2)

A 31-year-old man presents with episodic perianal pain for more than a year. He has occasionally noticed some discharge. On examination, a pit is seen in the lower natal cleft. It is filled with hair and a minimal amount of discharge is produced when pressure is applied to the region.

What is the most likely diagnosis?

A. Perianal abscess
B. Perianal haematoma
C. Pilonidal sinus
D. Proctalgia fugax
E. Rectal prolapse

40. MANAGING ARTERIAL DISEASE (1)

A 68-year-old man attends the emergency department following two episodes of weakness in the left side of his face, each lasting 2 hours. These resolve spontaneously and completely. Examination is unremarkable except for a left carotid bruit.

Which of the following steps would you take next?

A. Start aspirin, advise smoking cessation and refer for outpatient CT head
B. Start aspirin, advise smoking cessation and refer for outpatient carotid Doppler
C. Start aspirin and refer for urgent inpatient assessment
D. Start aspirin and refer to ophthalmology
E. Start steroids, advise smoking cessation and refer for CT head

41. SHOULDER DISORDERS (2)

A 65-year-old woman attends the GP practice. Yesterday, while gardening, she experienced sudden-onset pain in her right shoulder. On examination, there is some bruising of the upper arm, and on flexion of the elbow a bulge is seen in the upper arm.

Which of the following is the most likely diagnosis?

A. Distal rupture of biceps tendon
B. Proximal rupture of biceps tendon
C. Rotator cuff tear
D. Rupture of triceps
E. Supraspinatus tendonitis

42. LOIN PAIN

A 27-year-old man presents to the emergency department with a 2-hour history of severe left-sided loin pain which woke him from sleep. The pain is constant but occasionally dulls. He has been feeling sick with the pain and vomited twice. On examination, the patient is writhing in agony and has mild tenderness in the left loin only. His temperature is 36.9°C. Urine dipstick shows 2+ of blood.

What is the most likely diagnosis?

A. Biliary colic
B. Dissecting aortic aneurysm
C. Pyelonephritis
D. Renal cell carcinoma
E. Renal colic

43. DYSPHAGIA (2)

A 64-year-old woman presents to the GP complaining of pain and difficulty in swallowing. It is becoming progressively worse and now she complains it is even hard to drink water. On examination, she appears cachexic.

Which of the following is the most likely diagnosis?

A. Oesophageal candidiasis
B. Oesophageal carcinoma
C. Oesophageal spasm
D. Oesophageal stricture
E. Oesophageal web

44. PAEDIATRIC ORTHOPAEDICS (2)

An 8-year-old boy is brought in to the GP practice by his mother. He has been complaining of pain in his right hip for a few weeks and has started walking with a limp. Examination reveals limited range of movement at the hip. An X-ray of the pelvis shows a collapsed femoral head on the right.

What is the most likely diagnosis?

A. Femoral osteomyelitis
B. Perthes disease
C. Proximal femoral fracture
D. Slipped upper femoral epiphysis
E. Transient synovitis

45. FOOT DISORDERS (2)

A 32-year-old man presents to the GP with pain in the right foot which is exacerbated by weight bearing. He tells you he jogs on a daily basis. On examination, he has a tender swelling over the second metatarsal. An X-ray of his foot shows a periosteal reaction over the neck of the second metatarsal.

What is the most likely diagnosis?

A. Gout
B. Hallux rigidus
C. Jones fracture

D. Lisfranc fracture
E. March fracture

46. ULCERS (2)

A 62-year-old woman presents with a large painless, ulcerated lesion over her lower leg. It has been developing gradually over an area of scarring where she sustained a burn several years ago.
What is the most likely diagnosis?

A. Hypertrophic scars
B. Infected ulcer
C. Keloid scar
D. Marjolin ulcer
E. Perforated ulcer

47. THE SWOLLEN LIMB (2)

A 27-year-old woman presents to the GP with a 2-month history of worsening swelling in both legs. On examination, her lower legs and thighs are very oedematous and firm. The skin is thick, hard and grey in colour.
What is the most likely diagnosis?

A. Filariasis
B. Hereditary angioedema
C. Lymphoedema praecox
D. Lymphoedema tarda
E. Milroy disease

48. INVESTIGATING DYSPHAGIA (2)

A 56-year-old woman presents to the GP complaining of episodes of severe retrosternal chest pain after eating, associated with a bitter taste in her mouth. She has no difficulty or pain when swallowing. Examination is unremarkable.
Which of the following investigations would be most useful in establishing the cause of her symptoms?

A. 24-hour lower oesophageal pH
B. Barium swallow
C. Erect chest X-ray
D. Manometry
E. Upper gastrointestinal endoscopy

49. UPPER LIMB NERVE LESIONS (1)

The orthopaedic surgeon on call has been called down to the emergency department to see a patient who fractured his elbow 3 weeks ago and is suspected to have an ulnar nerve injury.

What would she expect to find on examination?

A. Complete paralysis of the forearm
B. Wasting of the hand, except the thenar eminence, and clawing of the ring and little fingers
C. Wasting of the thenar eminence and clawing of the index and middle fingers
D. Wasting of the thenar eminence with inability to abduct the thumb
E. Wrist drop and loss of sensation over the anatomical snuffbox

50. ABDOMINAL PAIN (6)

A 32-year-old woman who has been undergoing fertility treatment presents with a 2-hour history of right-sided lower abdominal pain, associated with nausea. On direct questioning she tells you she has had several similar, but less severe, episodes in the past. She has had no other genitourinary symptoms. Her pregnancy test is negative.

Which of the following is the most likely diagnosis?

A. Appendicitis
B. Ectopic pregnancy
C. Pelvic inflammatory disease
D. Torsion of the ovary
E. Urinary tract infection

Practice Paper 2: Answers

1. ABDOMINAL INCISIONS (1)

C – Right Kocher

A Kocher incision is made 3 cm below and parallel to the subcostal margin from the midline to the border of the rectus abdominus muscle. A right-sided Kocher incision is appropriate for an open cholecystectomy. Left-sided incisions are used for splenectomy. The incision cannot be extended medially, and if it is extended too far laterally, many intercostal nerves can be damaged. A rooftop incision (or double Kocher incision) is made up of both a left and a right Kocher incision connected at the middle. It provides good access to the liver and spleen. It is also indicated for use in bilateral adrenalectomy, radical pancreatic and gastric surgery.

The gridiron and Lanz incisions are used when doing an appendicectomy. The gridiron incision is made one-third of the way along, and at right angles to, the line connecting the anterior superior iliac spine to the umbilicus in the right iliac fossa (i.e. McBurney point). A Lanz incision is more transverse in orientation and closer to the anterior superior iliac spine when compared to the gridiron incision, and is made in the skin crease. A Lanz incision is preferred in younger girls as it provides a better cosmetic result. However, these incisions tend to divide the iliohypogastric and ilioinguinal nerves resulting in denervation of the muscles of the inguinal canal, increasing the risk of an inguinal hernia.

Paramedian incisions are made 1.5 cm from the midline through the rectus sheath. They have been used as an approach to gross abdominal surgery, in particular to visualize the kidneys and spleen, but are now avoided due to a poor cosmetic outcome.

Emil Theodore Kocher, Swiss surgeon (1841–1917).

Otto Lanz, Swiss surgeon (1865–1935).

2. SHOCK (2)

A – Antibiotics

Shock is a life-threatening condition in which there is *insufficient tissue perfusion, leading to inadequate oxygenation of organs*. If left untreated, this will result in multi-organ failure and death. The causes of shock may be broadly classified according to their aetiology into hypovolaemic, cardiogenic, anaphylactic, septic and neurogenic. This patient has presented in septic shock, where tissue hypoperfusion occurs secondary to marked systemic vasodilatation, induced by the inflammatory response. The most common cause of septic shock is endotoxin-producing Gram-negative bacilli. The mainstay of treatment, in addition to supportive measures, is systemic antibiotics. Antihistamines together with steroids and adrenaline are used in the treatment of anaphylactic shock, and atropine is used to treat the bradycardia of neurogenic shock. Inotropes increase myocardial contractility and can be used in the treatment of many types of shock including septic and cardiogenic. Intravenous fluids are used to treat the hypotension associated with most types of shock.

3. UPPER GI BLEED (2)

D – Mallory-Weiss tear

A Mallory-Weiss tear is a superficial mucosal tear. They occur most commonly at either the gastro-oesophageal junction or gastric cardia. Tears are caused by sudden increases in gastric pressure as occur with retching, repeated vomiting and coughing. Bleeding settles spontaneously within 48 hours in around 90% of cases and the tear heals within a fortnight. Diagnosis is confirmed at endoscopy. The treatment is largely supportive (resuscitation and proton pump inhibitors), unless active bleeding is seen on endoscopy (rare).

In contrast to a Mallory-Weiss tear, Boerhaave syndrome is a transluminal perforation of the oesophagus. Oesophageal varices are a cause of haematemesis in chronic alcohol abuse and develop secondary to portal hypertension caused by liver cirrhosis. Epistaxis is a nose bleed. If large amounts of blood are swallowed during a nose bleed, it may present as bloody vomiting or digested blood in the stools (melaena). Haemoptysis is the term given to blood which is coughed up, the origin of the blood being below the level of the larynx. Causes include pneumonia, pulmonary embolism and lung neoplasia.

Varices can occur in several places in the body, at the points of porto-systemic anastomosis (where the portal venous circulation anastomoses with the systemic venous circulation). All varices have the potential to bleed. The sites of porto-systemic anastomosis are oesophageal, rectal, paraumbilical, retroperitoneal and intrahepatic.

George Kenneth Mallory, American pathologist (1900–1986).

Soma Weiss, Hungarian physician (1898–1942).

4. BONE TUMOURS (2)

C – Ewing sarcoma

Ewing sarcoma is an extremely rare malignant tumour of bone that is most common in the 5–15-year age range. It is a small cell carcinoma that most commonly occurs in the legs or pelvis. Patients present with a painful swelling and fever. X-ray shows a lytic lesion with a laminated periosteal reaction, known as 'onion skinning'. Treatment is by neoadjuvant chemotherapy and/or radiotherapy with surgical excision.

A *chondrosarcoma* is a slow-growing malignant tumour of the cartilage that affects middle-aged patients. X-rays show localized bone destruction with areas of calcification within the tumour. Treatment is by chemotherapy with wide local excision. An *osteoid osteoma* is a benign, painful, self-limiting tumour of the bone that occurs in children and young adults. It presents with intense pain that is characteristically worse at night and is relieved by NSAIDs. Osteoid osteomas are caused by a nidus of osteoblasts that become trapped in the cortex of the bone. X-rays show a radiolucent nidus surrounded by a dense area of reactive bone. *Enchondromas* are common benign bone lesions of cartilaginous origin. They develop from aberrant cartilage left within a bone and are usually found in the metaphysis. Enchondromas are usually asymptomatic and are found incidentally. X-rays show a well-demarcated calcifying lesion within the metaphysis. Enchondromas can be single or multiple (Oilier disease).

James Ewing, American pathologist (1866–1943).

Louis Xavier Edouard Leopold Oilier, French surgeon (1830–1900).

5. BILIARY TRACT DISEASE (2)

B – Gallstone ileus
This patient has presented with the symptoms and signs of small bowel obstruction. Gallstone ileus is a rare cause of small bowel obstruction (5% of cases) but is most common in elderly women. It is not a true ileus in that the obstruction is not a result of bowel dysmotility but a mechanical obstruction caused by an impacted gallstone in the small bowel. Gallstone ileus occurs when a stone erodes through the gallbladder into the duodenum, forming a cholecysto-duodenal fistula. The most common site of impaction of the stone is at the ileocaecal junction. Gastric outlet obstruction caused by an impacted gallstone is known as Bouveret syndrome. Gallstones only usually cause a mechanical obstruction if they are large (>2.5 cm) or multiple. The classical radiological findings of Rigler's triad – small bowel obstruction + pneumobilia (air in the biliary tree, arising from the cholecysto-duodenal fistula) + ectopic gallstones as seen on abdominal X-ray, US or CT – make a definitive diagnosis. Treatment includes resuscitation and urgent surgical removal of the stone (laparotomy). There is a mortality rate of up to 20%.

Other causes of pneumobilia include emphysematous cholecystitis (caused by gas-forming organisms), pyogenic cholecystitis, post-ERCP, postcholecystectomy, blunt abdominal trauma and an incompetent sphincter of Oddi. Pneumobilia is not caused by a perforated gallbladder, though free air under the diaphragm may be seen on the erect chest X-ray.

Leon Bouveret, French physician (1850–1929).

Leo George Rigler, American radiologist (1896–1979).

6. CUTANEOUS MALIGNANCIES (2)

A – Basal cell carcinoma

Basal cell carcinoma (rodent ulcer) is the most common form of skin cancer and arises from the basal layer of the epidermis. It typically occurs on sun-exposed areas, although there is also a genetic predisposition to the condition. Various subtypes of basal cell carcinoma exist but the classic appearance is of a 'pearly' lesion with a rolled edge and telangiectasia. Basal cell carcinomas invade locally and rarely metastasize. The majority can be excised but, if too large, can be treated with radiotherapy, and if superficial, by topical chemotherapy (fluorouracil). Overall prognosis is good.

Seborrhoeic keratoses are common benign tumours also known as senile warts. They are flat pigmented lesions which grow to have a greasy 'stuck-on' appearance. Problems arise if they get stuck to clothes or become infected. The sign of Leser–Trélat is an acute eruption of multiple seborrhoeic keratoses that is associated with an underlying malignancy.

7. MANAGING ANORECTAL DISEASE (2)

C – Haemorrhoidectomy

Haemorrhoids are enlarged engorged vascular cushions within the rectum. They are common in Western populations and are associated with constipation, obesity and pregnancy. Haemorrhoids may be asymptomatic or present with a range of symptoms including pruritus, bleeding, soiling, a dragging sensation and pain, particularly if strangulated. They can be seen clearly on proctoscopy and are found at the 3, 7 and 11 o'clock positions with the patient in the lithotomy position. Haemorrhoids are graded as follows:

1. Do not prolapse
2. Prolapse on defaecation but spontaneously reduce
3. Reduce with manual reduction
4. Cannot be reduced

The treatment of minimally symptomatic piles includes stool softeners and a high fibre diet to prevent constipation. Local anaesthetic ointments may provide symptomatic relief. Small haemorrhoids (grades 1 and 2) can be treated with sclerotherapy, where an irritant is injected into the submucosa of the piles causing fibrosis and atrophy, or banding, where a band applied around the stalk of the pile causes atrophy and separation. Manual anal dilatation performed under general anaesthesia (Lord stretch) can be used as an adjunct to treatment but is now largely redundant due to the high risk of faecal incontinence. Haemorrhoidectomy is the excision of piles and is used in the treatment of higher grade piles, piles which persistently bleed and in patients with recurrent thrombosis.

Haemorrhoids, from Greek *haima* = blood + *rhoia* = to flow; 'likely to bleed'.

Piles, from Latin *pila* = balls.

8. INVESTIGATING ENDOCRINE DISEASE (2)

C – 24-hour urinary 5-hydroxyindole acetic acid

Carcinoid tumours are tumours of enterochromaffin cells of the ileum that secrete serotonin (5-hydroxytryptamine, or 5-HT). The 5-HT that these tumours secrete is carried from the bowel, via the portal vein, to the liver where it is harmlessly broken down. However, when carcinoid tumours metastasize to the liver, they can secrete 5-HT directly into the bloodstream, bypassing liver metabolism and resulting in the symptoms described in this question. The presence of carcinoid metastases in the liver that result in symptoms is known as carcinoid syndrome. Features of the carcinoid syndrome include paroxysmal flushing, diarrhoea, bronchospasm and abdominal pain precipitated by stress, alcohol and caffeine. The diagnosis of carcinoid syndrome is made by measuring 24-hour urinary 5-hydroxyindole acetic acid (5-HIAA), a breakdown product of serotonin. Management is by resection or, in widespread disease, symptomatic treatment with octreotide (a somatostatin analogue that inhibits 5-HT release). Carcinoid tumours are slow-growing so, even if disseminated disease is present, patients can live for many years.

9. HERNIAS (2)

A – Direct inguinal hernia

The inguinal canal is 4 cm long and passes downwards and medially from the deep inguinal ring (an inch above the midpoint of the inguinal ligament) to the superficial inguinal ring (an inch above the pubic tubercle).

Direct inguinal hernias protrude straight out of the abdominal wall through a weakened area of the transversalis fascia without travelling down the inguinal canal. The anatomic distinction between direct and indirect inguinal hernias is by their position relative to the inferior epigastric arteries. Direct inguinal hernias are found medial to the inferior epigastric arteries and indirect inguinal hernias are lateral to them. Direct inguinal hernias pass through Hesselbach's triangle, a landmark bounded by the rectus muscle medially, inferior epigastric vessels laterally and the inguinal ligament inferiorly. Their position in relation to the inferior epigastric arteries can only really be made at the time of surgery.

Direct inguinal hernias are always acquired and are bilateral in 12% of cases. Risk factors include smoking (due to increased coughing causing bouts of high intra-abdominal pressure), obesity, heavy lifting and damage to the ilioinguinal nerve (which contributes to the nerve supply of the anterior abdominal wall and can be damaged by incisions to the lower abdomen, such as those gaining access to the appendix). The neck of direct inguinal hernias is wide and thus rarely strangulates.

An *indirect hernia* is one that travels down the inguinal canal and into the scrotum. Indirect inguinal hernias are the most common type of hernias and occur most often in young, active men and premature babies (as the processus vaginalis is more likely to be patent). Indirect inguinal hernias are also more common on the right side, because the right testicle descends later and there is a greater incidence of failed closure of the processus vaginalis. On examination, the hernia lies above and medial to the pubic tubercle and may be observed to descend into the scrotum on standing or coughing. It does not transilluminate nor is the examiner able to palpate the upper border of the lump.

The femoral triangle is found on the upper thigh just below the inguinal ligament and contains, from lateral to medial, the femoral nerve, femoral artery and femoral vein (remember 'NAVY': Nerve, Artery, Vein, Y-fronts). The femoral canal is a space just medial to the femoral vein that contains fat, lymph nodes and vessels. It is in this potential space that femoral hernias can protrude. *Femoral hernias* are the third most common spontaneous hernia, occurring most frequently in older, multiparous women (this is because the femoral ring is bigger in females and pregnancy stretches the fascia over the femoral canal). They protrude through the narrow femoral ring and into the femoral canal where they expand considerably. On examination, femoral hernias are below and lateral to the pubic tubercle and the right side is affected twice as commonly as the left. Because the neck of the femoral ring is narrow there is a high risk of strangulation (50% at 1 month), thus all femoral hernias should be operated on urgently.

Franz Hesselbach, German surgeon and anatomist (1759–1816).

10. GROIN LUMPS (2)

B – Hydrocele

A hydrocele is a collection of serous fluid in the tunica vaginalis, a membrane that covers the testis. They can be primary or secondary to an underlying cause. Primary hydroceles (as in this case) are tense, painless, fluctuant swellings which transilluminate. They are commoner in boys. Because the fluid surrounds the testicle, the underlying testis is not palpable, however the epididymis above can be felt as a separate structure and you are able to feel the upper border of the swelling (this would *not* be the case with a hernia). Primary hydroceles are benign but can be surgically excised if desired. (Simple aspiration of the cyst will result in re-accumulation of fluid.) A secondary hydrocele can occur when the membranous sac around the testis becomes filled with exudates secondary to tumours or inflammation of the underlying testis or epididymis. Secondary hydroceles are usually small and lax.

Hydroceles in adults should be investigated with ultrasound to exclude underlying pathology. If no serious pathology is found, treatment can be with scrotal supports, aspiration of fluid or open surgery if there is a large or recurrent hydrocele. Testicular torsion and epididymo-orchitis both present with acute testicular pain and marked tenderness on examination.

The term *varicocele* describes varicosities in the pampiniform venous plexus, the network of veins that drains the testicle. It usually occurs on the left side and is present in 10% of males. Patients present with a scrotal swelling on standing that feels like a 'bag of worms' and may experience a heavy, dragging sensation. Varicoceles are usually harmless but have been associated with defective spermatogenesis rendering some patients subfertile (although this is a contentious issue). Varicoceles can be diagnosed by ultrasound, which shows venous dilatation greater than 2 mm. Management is by reassurance and advising the wearing of supportive underwear. If a patient desires treatment then radiological embolization of the left testicular vein, or ligation and division of the testicular veins, can be performed.

In some cases a left-sided varicocele can be indicative of left renal pathology due to impaired venous drainage secondary to a renal mass causing increased backpressure.

11. BREAST DISEASE (2)

C – Fibroadenoma

Fibroadenomas are common breast lumps that most frequently occur in women aged 15–25 years. They present as discrete, firm, freely mobile lumps, 2–3 cm in size, which classically 'slip' under the examining fingers. For this reason, they are also known as 'breast mice'. Excision of the lesions is not required as there is no risk of malignancy and most resolve over a period of years.

Breast cysts typically present as a sudden, painful swelling in the breast. They are most common in the forties. Diagnosis and treatment is by aspiration, which reveals a clear fluid. In 30% of cases breast cysts recur – these require surgical excision. Occasionally breast cyst aspirate is blood-stained and this is suggestive of malignancy within the wall of the cyst. If this is the case, local excision of the lesion is required.

Bacterial mastitis describes infection of a lactiferous duct by *Staphylococcus aureus,* which is transmitted by an infant's nasopharynx during lactation. It presents with cellulitis around the infected area with pyrexia, tachycardia and a leukocytosis. A complication of bacterial mastitis is the formation of a *breast abscess,* resulting in a palpable lump.

The mainstay of treatment of bacterial mastitis is antibiotics. However if an abscess is present it must be aspirated or drained.

Gynaecomastia is the benign proliferation of male breast tissue due to an imbalance of oestrogens and androgens. It is physiological (normal) in neonates, puberty and in the elderly. There are many other causes of gynaecomastia; these include drugs (cimetidine, spironolactone, cannabis, oestrogen, steroids), renal failure, cirrhosis and testicular tumours. Obesity is not a cause of true gynaecomastia. Although most cases of gynaecomastia resolve spontaneously, excision can be offered if lesions do not settle or are symptomatic or embarrassing. Most commonly, male gynaecomastia can be painful in older men on hormone deprivation therapy for prostate cancer.

Phyllodes tumours (a.k.a. cystosarcoma phyllodes) are rare tumours of the fibroepithelial stroma of the breast, accounting for <1% of all breast tumours. They are typically benign but fast-growing, and have a distinctive leaf-like appearance on histology.

Gynaecomastia, from Latin *gynae* = woman + *mastia* = breast.

Phyllodes, from Greek *phullon* = leaf; these tumours have a leaf-like appearance on histology.

12. PAEDIATRIC SURGICAL MANAGEMENT (2)

A – Barium enema

This child has presented with features of intussusception. Intussusception is a condition in which one part of the bowel (the intussusceptum) invaginates into the adjacent distal segment of bowel (the intussuscipiens). Invagination leads to compression of the mesentery with venous engorgement leading to oedema and ischaemia which, if left untreated, will result in necrotic bowel, gastrointestinal haemorrhage, perforation, peritonitis, septicaemia and death. The most common site of intussusception is the junction between the terminal ileum and caecum. The cause is unknown in the majority of cases but an increased risk is observed with recent upper respiratory tract infections (believed to be secondary to enlarged lymph nodes), Henoch-Schönlein purpura (purpuric haemorrhages in the bowel provide the focus for an intussusception), Meckel diverticulum and intestinal polyps. Intussusception is most common between the ages of 6 and 9 months and is the leading cause of obstruction in children up to the age of 6 years. It is much more common in boys. Children typically present with paroxysmal episodes of colicky abdominal pain, with drawing up of the legs towards the abdomen. Initially the child is well in between episodes. There may be associated vomiting and diarrhoea, and the passage of 'red-currant jelly' stools (bloody mucus) per rectum occurs late in the condition. A sausage-shaped mass may be palpable in the right upper quadrant. Fever is only present in the presence of necrosis and sepsis. If the diagnosis of intussusception is suspected then a contrast enema must be performed as soon as possible following resuscitation. A barium enema not only establishes the diagnosis but may successfully reduce the intussusception (in 80%). Recurrence may occur in up to 10%. If there is any indication of perforation or peritonitis, or the enema is unsuccessful, a laparotomy must be performed.

13. ARTERIAL BLOOD GASES (2)

C – Fully compensated respiratory acidosis

This woman presents with features highly suggestive of bronchial malignancy, and is most probably a smoker. The blood gas shows a normal pH, but on the acidotic side, with a high pCO_2 and high bicarbonate. She therefore has a fully compensated respiratory acidosis (as well as a type II respiratory failure, as the pO_2 is less than 8). Note that this is not a venous sample because the saturations on the blood gas correspond to what was recorded on the monitor – in a venous sample the blood gas saturations would be well below that of the pulse oximeter.

See the question 'Arterial blood gases (1)' for further information on interpreting arterial blood gas results.

14. JAUNDICE (2)

B – Ascending cholangitis

Ascending cholangitis is caused by bacterial infection of the biliary tract, as a result of bile stasis secondary to obstruction. Typical offending organisms are *E. coli* and *Klebsiella*. Presentation is with severe colicky right upper quadrant pain, fevers and rigors, and jaundice (Charcot's triad). These three features, along with hypotension and confusion, make up Reynolds' pentad of symptoms. Resuscitation and administration of intravenous antibiotics must be prompt as septicaemia can occur rapidly. Biliary drainage is also required. Ascending cholangitis has a mortality of at least 5%.

Biliary colic presents as pain alone without systemic upset or change in blood markers. Treatment is symptomatic and pain usually resolves within 24 hours.

Acute cholecystitis is inflammation of the gallbladder and there are no associated obstructive features. *Gallstone ileus* is caused by erosion of gallstones into the duodenum and presents with features of bowel obstruction. It is more common in elderly patients. *Carcinoma of the gallbladder* is rare, but associated with gallstones in 80% of cases. Its presentation is more insidious and a palpable mass may be found in the right upper quadrant.

Jean-Marie Charcot, French neurologist (1825–1893).

15. PREOPERATIVE MORBIDITY (2)

B – ASA grade II

For an explanation of ASA grading, please see the question 'Preoperative morbidity (1)'.

16. THYROID DISEASE (2)

A – De Quervain thyroiditis

De Quervain thyroiditis describes transient inflammation of the thyroid gland associated with viral infection. It is the most common cause of a painful thyroid gland and is typically seen in the younger, female patient. The clinical course of de Quervain thyroiditis is highly variable and in the initial stages there may be features of hyperthyroidism. This usually resolves spontaneously. Following this, there may be a period of hypo-thyroidism, which can become permanent in 10% of cases. Treatment is largely symptomatic, with anti-inflammatories, and thyroid dysfunction can be treated on a short-term basis.

Riedel thyroiditis is a rare condition in which normal thyroid tissue is replaced by dense fibrous tissue which may extend beyond the gland, causing dysphagia and tracheal compression. Hypothyroidism develops in 30% of cases. Presentation is with a painless 'fixed' goitre and may mimic carcinoma of the thyroid. The diagnosis is confirmed histologically following biopsy. Surgical treatment is required if there are compressive symptoms. A third of patients develop fibrosis at other sites including the lacrimal gland and lung. *Hashimoto thyroiditis* is an autoimmune con-dition largely affecting women and caused by circulating autoantibod-ies to peroxidise thyroglobulin. It is a common cause of hypothyroidism although there may be an initial phase of hyperthyroidism. The thyroid gland is enlarged, firm and non-tender. Treatment is with levothyroxine. A *thyroglossal cyst* is a persistence of the thyroglossal duct from the descent of the thyroid at the base of the tongue. These cysts are found in the mid-line of the neck and characteristically move upwards on protrusion of the tongue. Symptoms arise if the cyst enlarges or becomes infected.

Hakari Hashimoto, Japanese surgeon (1881–1934).

Fritz de Quervain, Swiss surgeon (1868–1940).

Bernhard Moritz Riedel, German surgeon (1846–1916).

17. ABDOMINAL PAIN (4)

E – Perforated peptic ulcer

A perforated peptic ulcer is a life-threatening surgical emergency in which complete erosion of a pre-existing peptic ulcer leads to the spillage of stomach contents into the peritoneum. This causes a chemical peritoni-tis which, if untreated, becomes a bacterial peritonitis. Perforated ulcers are most common in middle-aged men but a larger number of cases are being seen in elderly women secondary to NSAID use. The majority of those who present with perforation would have had symptoms of peptic ulcer disease. Most perforations occur in the duodenum; perforation of stomach ulcers is associated with gastric carcinoma in a third of cases. Presentation is much less acute in a posterior gastric ulcer perforation, as spillage is into, and contained within, the lesser sac. Other features of a perforated peptic ulcer are haematemesis and melaena. Endoscopy is contraindicated in the presence of a perforation, however, due to the risk of exacerbating gastric leakage into the peritoneum. Free air is often seen under the diaphragm in an erect chest X-ray, although its absence does not exclude a perforation (free air is not seen in at least 10% of cases). Occasionally, free air not seen on an AP view may be detected on a lateral decubitus film. If perforation is suspected, urgent resuscitation of the patient is required, with the administration of intravenous fluids and intravenous proton pump inhibitors, prior to transfer to theatre. Perforations may become sealed by overlying omentum; these cases may be treated conservatively. The mortality of perforated peptic ulcers increases with age and is up to 10%. Consider testing patients with peptic ulceration for *H. pylori* infection.

Other causes of air under the diaphragm, other than the perforation of a hollow viscus, include post-abdominal surgery, lung pathology (e.g. fistulae) and penetrating trauma.

18. FLUID THERAPY (1)

D – 2400 mL

In any adult who is estimated to have 15% of burns or more, and in any child who has 10% or more, it is vital to initiate fluid replacement. Burns result in increased capillary permeability with fluid loss which, with extensive burn areas, can result in hypovolaemic shock. The majority of fluid loss with burns injury occurs in the first 12 hours, but continues for up to 36 hours. Various formulae are used to assess the amount of fluid required for resuscitation.

One of the widely used formulas is the Muir and Barclay (a.k.a. Mount Vernon Burns Unit) formula, which states that the amount of fluid to be given in any *period* (in mL) is calculated as follows:

$$\text{Fluid per } period \text{ (mL)} = \text{weight (kg)} \times \% \text{ burn area}/2$$

The *periods* are as follows:

	Every 4 hours for the first 12 hours
then	*Every* 6 hours for the next 12 hours
then	Over 12 hours for the next 12 hours

Thus, six volumes are given *over* the first 36 hours. Note that this is in addition to the patient's normal fluid replacement.

As the fluid lost in burns is of a similar composition to plasma, a combination of colloid (e.g. Gelofusine) and crystalloid (e.g. Hartmann) would be appropriate. If burns are full thickness, 50% of the fluid should be blood, to replace the red cell destruction that occurs in the burn. Fluid replacement must start from the time the burn occurred, not the time of arrival of the patient – if the *above* patient arrived in hospital an hour following burns injury, the first ration of fluid must be given *over* 3 hours. Haemodynamic markers and urine output can be used to monitor the response to fluid replacement.

19. ENDOCRINE DISEASE (2)

D – Multiple endocrine neoplasia type IIb

This young patient has features of a phaeochromocytoma. This, along with his history of thyroid cancer and a marfanoid phenotype (tall + arachnodactyly), suggests a diagnosis of multiple endocrine neoplasia (MEN) type IIb.

There are three types of MEN, all of which are autosomal dominant conditions. MEN type I (Wermer syndrome) includes the presence of parathyroid adenomas, pancreatic islet-cell tumours and pituitary adenomas. MEN type IIa (Sipple syndrome) comprises parathyroid adenomas, medullary carcinoma of the thyroid and phaeochromocytoma. Finally MEN type IIb (more recently renamed as MEN type III) includes the presence of the tumours of MEN type IIa but with the addition of multiple mucosal neuromas of the gastrointestinal tract and a marfanoid phenotype.

Paul Wermer, American physician (1898–1975).

John Sipple, American physician (1930–present).

20. MANAGING ABDOMINAL PAIN (2)

B – Omeprazole, clarithromycin and metronidazole

This patient has peptic ulcer disease associated with *Helicobacter pylori* infection, as determined by a positive urease test (Campylobacter-like organism [CLO] test). Eighty percent of peptic ulcers are associated with *H. pylori* infection. *H. pylori* is a Gram-negative, spiral-shaped rod that can colonize gastric-type mucosa, whether that be in the stomach itself or gastric-type metaplasia in the oesophagus or duodenum. Infection is found in 50% of the over-50s, but most people with it are asymptomatic. *H. pylori* produces urease, an enzyme that converts urea into ammonia. The ammonia it releases neutralizes the acidic pH around it, which is why this bacterium can live in the harsh acidic environment of the stomach. *H. pylori* damages gastric mucosa by releasing toxic ammonia and cytokines as well as by increasing stomach acid secretion by stimulating gastrin production. The ability of *H. pylori* to convert urea into ammonia by action of the enzyme urease is the basis of the rapid urease test (or CLO test). Other ways of detecting the presence of *H. pylori* include the urease breath test and the stool antigen test. The combination of peptic ulceration with concurrent *H. pylori* infection is an indication for triple therapy: a proton pump inhibitor with clarithromycin and metronidazole. This is usually given for one week. Repeat testing can confirm the eradication of *H. pylori*. Biopsies can also be taken at the time of endoscopy if gastric ulceration as a consequence of *H. pylori* is suspected.

Non-steroidal anti-inflammatory drugs are the second most common cause of peptic ulceration. They inhibit the synthesis of prostaglandins by inhibiting the action of cycle-oxygenase (COX) which is protective of the gastric mucosa. There are two forms of COX: type 1 and type 2. Type 2 has less effect on the gastric mucosa and therefore selective COX2 inhibitors, e.g. celecoxib, carry a smaller risk of peptic ulceration than non-selective COX inhibitors. Notably, however, they may confer an increased risk of myocardial infarction.

There is also an association between long-term steroid use and peptic ulceration; therefore in those taking either of these drugs on a regular long-term basis it may be sensible to add a proton pump inhibitor to reduce the risk of ulceration. Ranitidine, a histamine-2 receptor antagonist, is used for the symptomatic relief of peptic ulceration and gastro-oesophageal reflux.

Peptic ulcers are four times more likely to develop in the duodenum than the stomach. All gastric ulcers must be biopsied due to their potential for malignant change (unlike duodenal ulcers).

21. SKIN LESIONS (2)

A – Cavernous haemangioma

A cavernous haemangioma (or strawberry naevus) is a condition that appears in the first months of life as a bright red lesion on the face or trunk that grows rapidly. Occasionally these lesions bleed or ulcerate. Cavernous haemangiomas eventually regress and disappear spontaneously, so intervention is only required if lesions persist beyond a few years of age. Cavernous haemangiomas may rarely be associated with thrombocytopenia and haemolytic anaemia secondary to trapping and destruction of platelets and erythrocytes within the lesions. This is known as Kasabach-Merritt syndrome.

A *deep capillary naevus* (or port-wine stain) is a malformation of the capillaries in the deep and superficial dermis. These are congenital malformations which can occur anywhere in the body but are most often found unilaterally on the face. Occasionally a port-wine stain is associated with seizures, mental retardation and eye abnormalities (glaucoma, optic atrophy) due to underlying cranial malformations. This is known as *Sturge-Weber syndrome* and is usually associated with a port-wine stain in the distribution of the ophthalmic or maxillary division of the trigeminal nerve.

A *superficial capillary naevus* (or salmon patch) is a small, flat, pink patch of skin with poorly defined borders. It is commonly found on the forehead (angel's kiss) or on the nape of the neck (stork mark). Most superficial naevi disappear in the first year of life.

Trigeminal, from Latin *tri* = three + *gemini* = twins; which together means 'triplets'.

The trigeminal nerve has three divisions.

Haig Kasabach, American paediatrician (1898–1943).

Katherine Merritt, American paediatrician (1886–1986).

William Allen Sturge, English physician (1850–1919).

Frederick Parkes Weber, English physician (1863–1962).

22. NECK LUMPS (2)

B – Cystic hygroma

A cystic hygroma is a congenital benign proliferation of lymph vessels that is found in the posterior triangle of the neck. It is a multi-cystic swelling that is fleshy and compressible and contains clear fluid. Cystic hygromas characteristically transilluminate 'brightly'. Diagnosis is confirmed by CT or MRI and treatment is by excision of the mass.

The posterior triangle of the neck is bounded by the sternocleidomastoid muscle in front, the anterior border of trapezius behind and the middle third of the clavicle at its base. The apex of the triangle is the occiput.

Hygroma, from Greek *hygros* = wet + *oma* = tumour; so-called because it contains fluid.

23. CONDITIONS OF THE NOSE

E – Refer to ENT on call to remove foreign body

It is a common occurrence for children to insert foreign bodies into the nose and, after recovering from the initial trauma, forget that it is there! The foreign body is usually found anterior to the middle turbinate. A foreign body in the nostril can result in chronic inflammation, presenting with a foul-smelling, blood-stained purulent discharge. Complications of intranasal foreign bodies include respiratory compromise, aspiration and localized infection which can potentially spread (e.g. meningitis). Rarely a foreign body may present with myiasis (infestation of tissue with fly larvae – maggots!). It is important therefore to remove intranasal foreign bodies; however this must be done by an experienced clinician as there is risk of causing further mucosal damage and pushing the object further into the nasal passage. Removal must be carried out under appropriate sedation (topical lidocaine) with the child appropriately restrained and with the foreign body under direct visualization. Phenylephrine is often administered intranasally to reduce oedema and bleeding. A variety of techniques may be used to remove objects, including forceps and suction.

Attempts can be made to expel the object by pressing on the contralateral nostril and asking the child to blow through the nose forcefully.

Nasal packing is used in cases where epistaxis is not controlled by direct pressure and is contraindicated here as it would force the object further into the nose. Cauterization may be chemical (silver nitrate) or electrical and is a treatment option in severe epistaxis.

24. ABDOMINAL PAIN (5)

D – Pelvic inflammatory disease

Acute pelvic inflammatory disease (PID) is caused by ascending infection from the vagina or cervix causing inflammation of the upper reproductive tract. It commonly presents in young women and affects 2% of women in their lifetime. PID is usually caused by sexually transmitted infections, such as *Chlamydia trachomatis* and *Neisseria gonorrhoeae* (>80% of cases), but may also be caused iatrogenically, e.g. by insertion of intra-uterine devices and following termination of pregnancy. Presenting features include lower abdominal pain, deepdyspareunia, dysuria and vaginal discharge. Diagnosis is made by taking vaginal and cervical swabs, but treatment with appropriate antibiotics is commenced immediately to reduce the risk of long-term damage. A typical antibiotic regimen includes 2 weeks of ofloxacin (anti-chlamydia and gonorrhoea) and metronidazole (anti-anaerobes and protozoa). If there is significant systemic upset, antibiotics are administered intravenously. Approximately 20% of women have recurrence of PID. Complications are largely secondary to adhesions and include ectopic pregnancy and infertility. Some women also develop Fitz-Hugh–Curtis syndrome – right upper quadrant pain caused by inflammation of the connective tissue around the liver by the pelvic infection.

Mittelschmerz is the name given to the lower abdominal pain that occurs during the middle of the menstrual cycle. It corresponds with ovulation. Mittelschmerz pains are benign and experienced by at least 20% of women. Treatment is with simple analgesia.

Remember that in any woman of child-bearing age presenting with abdominal pain, a pregnancy test must be carried out, so as not to miss an ectopic pregnancy.

Chlamydia, from Greek *chlamys* = cloak (as chlamydia is often 'cloaked', i.e. asymptomatic).

Mittelschmerz, from German *mittel* = middle + *schmerz* = pain ('pain that occurs mid-cycle').

Thomas Fitz-Hugh Jr, American physician (1894–1963).

Arthur Curtis, American gynaecologist (1881–1955).

25. COMPLICATIONS OF COLLES FRACTURES

E – Sudeck atrophy

A Colles fracture is a fracture of the distal radius within 2.5 cm of the wrist, associated with dorsal displacement and angulation of the distal fragment. Sudeck atrophy is a *reflex sympathetic dystrophy* that can affect any limb after injury and can occur in up to 30% of people with Colles fracture. It presents with a persistent burning pain associated with redness, swelling and warmth of the affected limb, which in the later stages can become pale and atrophied. Due to sympathetic stimulation there may be excessive sweating over this area. Active treatment with physiotherapy is required in the first instance. Carpal tunnel syndrome is caused by compression of the median nerve at the wrist and causes pain and numbness over the medial three and a half fingers with no skin changes. Compartment syndrome would be a much earlier complication of a fracture, usually caused by swelling within a tight plaster cast. Extensor pollicis longus rupture is caused by repetitive trauma over a bony fragment or by local ischaemia, and would result in the patient not being able to lift the thumb when the hand is placed flat on a table. Malunion would result in persistent deformity of the wrist.

Paul Herman Martin Sudeck, German surgeon (1866–1945).
Abraham Colles, Irish surgeon (1773–1843).

26. KNEE INJURIES

A – Positive Lachman test

Injury to the knee associated with an acute haemarthrosis is typical of a cruciate ligament injury. The knee contains two cruciate ligaments: the anterior, which prevents forward displacement of the tibia relative to the femur; and the posterior, which prevents backward displacement. Their integrity may be investigated using the Lachman test. Here the knee is kept flexed between 20 and 30 degrees and the tibia is pulled forward with the examiner sitting on the patient's foot. Increased movement in the anterior posterior direction (by more than 4 mm) is described as a positive test and is indicative of anterior cruciate ligament damage. A variation of this test with the knee flexed to 90 degrees is known as the 'anterior draw test'. The collateral ligaments are assessed with the knee flexed to 30 degrees; valgus and then varus stress is applied to the joint to assess the integrity of the lateral and medial collateral ligaments respectively. Excessive opening up of the joint is seen with collateral ligament injuries. The McMurray test is used to determine meniscal injuries. With the knee flexed to 90 degrees, lateral pressure is applied to the joint and the lower leg is externally rotated. Pain or palpable crepitus is indicative of a lateral meniscal injury. When medial pressure is applied to the joint and the lower leg is internally rotated, pain indicates a medial meniscal injury. The patellar apprehension test is used to assess the 'dislocatability' of the patella by applying pressure to it. The test is positive if the patient feels anxious that the knee cap is 'going to pop out'. The Simmonds (or Thompson) test is used to test the integrity of the Achilles tendon (the patient lies face down on the bed with the feet hanging off the edge – if there is no plantarflexion of the foot when squeezing the calf, then the test is positive for likely Achilles tendon rupture).

Franklin Adin Simmonds, English orthopaedic surgeon (1911–1983).

27. CHEST TRAUMA (2)

A – Analgesia and respiratory support

The cause of this patient's respiratory distress is a flail chest. A flail chest is a life-threatening injury caused by high impact trauma resulting in two or more consecutive ribs being broken in two or more places. That segment of the chest wall then moves independently, moving in on inspiration and out on expiration – 'paradoxical motion' (i.e. the opposite of what the remainder of the intact chest wall is doing). Flail chests are almost invariably associated with an underlying pulmonary contusion and there is a risk of pneumothorax from rupture of the pleura by bone ends. This injury is associated with a high mortality. It is important to make the patient comfortable, provide adequate analgesia such as intercostal nerve blocks (to encourage respiratory effort), and provide respiratory support. Depending on the degree of hypoxia, positive pressure ventilation may be required and its use has largely superseded rib fracture fixation. The mortality associated with a flail chest is largely dependent on the degree of the underlying pulmonary contusion.

Needle thoracocentesis is performed in the treatment of a tension pneumothorax.

28. EYE DISEASE (2)

E – Herpes simplex keratitis

Herpes simplex keratitis is a common but serious infection of the cornea caused by the herpes simplex virus. It most commonly presents in adult men many years after primary infection with the herpes simplex virus, where the virus lays dormant in the trigeminal nerve. It presents with a painful, watering, light-sensitive red eye and there may be a 'scratchy' sensation. The detection of a branch-like lesion – the 'dendritic ulcer' which contains live virus – is pathognomonic of this condition. Herpes simplex keratitis is treated with topical aciclovir until the ulcer has healed. There is a risk of corneal scarring and blindness so this condition warrants urgent ophthalmological assessment. Steroids are contraindicated as immunosuppression can lead to increased viral replication and the formation of a larger ulcer.

A *corneal abrasion* is caused by trauma, e.g. a scratch from a contact lens or foreign body. It presents with pain, photophobia, watering and the sensation of a foreign body in the eye. They are seen clearly after fluorescein staining. Corneal abrasions generally heal spontaneously within a few days. Topical antibiotics are generally prescribed to prevent concurrent infection.

Anterior uveitis (or iritis) presents with acute-onset eye pain, photophobia, blurred vision and lacrimation. On examination, there is likely to be circumcorneal redness, a small irregular pupil and decreased visual acuity. A layer of yellow exudate may be seen in the anterior chamber of the eye (hypopyon). In anterior uveitis the eye pain increases as the eyes converge and the pupils constrict. Anterior uveitis occurs in middle-aged and young adults and is associated with HLA-B27 joint problems (e.g. ankylosing spondylitis) and Behçet disease. Treatment is with topical steroids and atropine drops (to keep the pupils dilated and prevent adhesions from forming).

Episcleritis describes inflammation of the episclera, a thin membrane that covers the sclera. Episcleritis presents with painless reddening of the eye. It is common with autoimmune conditions, such as rheumatoid arthritis. On examination, dilated blood vessels will be seen only in the superficial layer of the sclera. Steroid eye drops provide symptomatic relief and aid recovery. *Conjunctivitis* presents with reddening and inflammation of the eye, along with lacrimation, itching and burning. Conjunctivitis can be allergic, viral or bacterial. Viral conjunctivitis often results in a watery discharge. Bacterial conjunctivitis is associated with a purulent discharge and is commonly caused by *Staphylococcus* or *Streptococcus* species. Many cases resolve spontaneously, but chloramphenicol eye drops hasten the response.

Sjögren syndrome is an autoimmune condition where antibodies act against secretory glands of the body resulting in 'dryness', including xerostomia (dry mouth) and keratoconjunctivitis sicca (ocular dryness), together known as the sicca symptoms.

29. HEPATOMEGALY (2)

D – Metastatic liver disease

This patient has presented with symptoms suggestive of lung cancer. It is likely that the cause of his hepatomegaly is metastatic spread of the cancer. The majority of malignant tumours of the liver are metastatic (secondary tumours), spreading from the lung, breast, gastrointestinal tract and prostate. Tumour deposits are often large and multiple giving a 'craggy' liver. Haematological malignancies such as leukaemia may also infiltrate the liver and present with hepatomegaly, although here the liver would be homogenously enlarged.

Hepatocellular carcinoma is the most common primary malignancy of the liver (90%). The majority of cases arise from a background of liver cirrhosis (e.g. alcohol, hepatitis B). Other causes include exposure to aflatoxins (toxins made by the fungus *Aspergillus,* which is found in soil and in grains) and schistosomiasis. Presentations include jaundice, ascites and nodular, painful hepatomegaly. Hepatocellular carcinoma is associated with the tumour marker alpha-fetoprotein. Diagnosis is easily confirmed with appropriate imaging (ultrasound or CT). The prognosis is poor (average survival being less than 6 months). Curative options include resection of the tumour or a liver transplant.

Budd-Chiari syndrome is characterized by the triad of abdominal pain, hepatomegaly and ascites caused by venous flow obstruction secondary to thrombosis of the hepatic vein (note: not the hepatic portal vein). Risk factors include thrombophilias, malignancy, trauma and the oral contraceptive pill. Diagnosis may be made on Doppler ultrasound scanning and venography. Treatment includes addressing the underlying cause, thrombolysis and surgery. A *Riedel lobe* is a tongue-like projection extending from the inferior border of the right side of the liver. It is a normal anatomical variant which may be mistaken for a pathologically enlarged liver or renal mass.

George Budd, English physician (1808–1882).

Hans Chiari, Austrian pathologist (1851–1916).

Bernhard Moritz Carl Ludwig Riedel, German surgeon (1846–1916).

30. NIPPLE DISCHARGE (2)

B – Duct ectasia

In duct ectasia, the mammary ducts dilate and fill with a stagnant greeny-brown 'cheesy' secretion. This fluid may discharge from the nipple and irritate the surrounding areola skin ('periductal mastitis'). Fibrosis of the duct eventually occurs, leading to nipple retraction. This condition is much commoner in smokers. On examination, a subareolar mass (the dilated, filled ducts) may be palpable. Management is by stopping smoking and surgical excision of the major ducts (Hadfield procedure).

31. PAEDIATRIC SURGERY (2)

B – Duodenal atresia

Duodenal atresia describes a complete obliteration of the duodenal lumen which occurs during embryonic development. It presents within the first 24 hours of life with bile-stained vomiting. It has an incidence of 1/6000 and affects males and females alike. There is an association with trisomy 21 (Down syndrome). Due to intestinal obstruction, the fetus is not able to swallow amniotic fluid, resulting in polyhydramnios. Diagnosis is confirmed by the presence of a double-bubble sign on the abdominal X-ray. This represents the presence of air in the stomach and proximal duodenum only, and not in the distal intestines. Definitive surgery in the neonatal period is required (duodeno-duodenostomy).

Choledochal cysts are a congenital abnormality of the bile ducts and may show a similar bubble appearance on imaging. However they do not result in polyhydramnios. *Oesophageal atresia* does cause polyhydramnios and presents in the neonatal period with excessive drooling and an inability to swallow. A chest X-ray is the first line of investigation. *Renal agenesis* (failure of development of the kidneys) results in oligohydramnios (deficiency of amniotic fluid) rather than polyhydramnios.

32. INVESTIGATING ABDOMINAL PAIN (2)

A – CT abdomen
Possible causes of this patient's pain include renal calculi, leaking abdominal aortic aneurysm, cholecystitis and a slipped intervertebral disc. His pain appears to be typical of renal colic, radiating from back to front; however, beware of making a first diagnosis of renal colic in the elderly, especially in a patient with known atherosclerotic disease. Rupturing abdominal aortic aneurysms can present in the same way. Therefore, as the patient is otherwise stable, it is safer to get a CT of the abdomen which would pick up either pathology instead of wasting time with an intravenous urogram. CT–KUB (kidney, ureter, bladder) is the gold standard investigation for diagnosing renal stones.

An ultrasound is not indicated as he is known to have gallstones; however, the normal inflammatory markers would not suggest cholecystitis. If this patient was haemodynamically unstable, urgent resuscitation and laparotomy would be indicated.

33. VASCULAR DISEASE (2)

D – Subclavian steal syndrome
This man has a cervical rib which is impinging on his right subclavian artery. When the arm is exerted it requires more blood but, because the subclavian artery is narrowed, the blood has to come from elsewhere. Instead it is 'stolen' from the vertebral artery which is meant to supply the brain. This is why, in cases of subclavian artery impingement, when the arm is over-used and blood is diverted away from the vertebral artery, a transient loss of consciousness occurs. This is known as the subclavian steal syndrome.

34. LOWER LIMB NERVE LESIONS (2)

C – Sciatic nerve
The sciatic nerve can be damaged with fracture dislocations of the hip or by misplaced gluteal injections. Sciatic nerve palsy results in paralysis of the hamstrings and all the muscles of the leg and foot. Sensation is lost below the knee except for the medial leg (supplied by the saphenous nerve, a branch of the femoral nerve) and the upper calf (supplied by the posterior femoral cutaneous nerve).

Sciatic, from Latin *sciaticus* = hip.

35. INVESTIGATING UROLOGICAL DISEASE (2)

D – Urethrography

This patient has presented with obstructive urinary symptoms, the likely cause being a urethral stricture. Urethral strictures are most commonly caused iatrogenically, e.g. during catheterization and instrumentation, but can also be caused by inflammation secondary to infections such as gonorrhoea and nonspecific urethritis. Balanitis xerotica obliterans is a scarring disease of the glans and foreskin which can extend up the urethra and cause troublesome urethral strictures at its advanced stage. Some strictures may be congenital in origin. Urethrography – in which a dye is inserted through the distal end of the meatus – is most useful in diagnosing strictures, as well as determining their length and number. Urinary flow rates will show an obstructive picture but will not necessarily be specific to the diagnosis of a stricture. If the stricture has been causing significant obstruction, renal ultrasound scan would show bilateral hydronephrosis, as would an intravenous urogram. The patient would also have a high post-void residual volume due to incomplete bladder emptying. Urethral strictures can be treated by dilatation, urethrotomy (incision made in the stricture), and in severe cases, urethroplasty (complete excision and repair of the narrowed urethra, with or without use of a tissue graft). Diversion surgery can also be performed, which would commonly take the form of a suprapubic catheter.

36. SPINAL CORD LESIONS (2)

A – Anterior cord syndrome

In general, the spinal cord is made up of three tracts on either side. A useful, simplified model of the spinal cord is as follows: the spinothalamic tract makes up the anterior third of the spinal cord and provides pain and temperature fibres to the contralateral side. The corticospinal tract is the middle third of the spinal cord and provides motor fibres to the ipsilateral side. Finally, the dorsal columns are found along the posterior length of the spinal cord and provide vibration sense and proprioception to the ipsilateral side.

The anterior cord syndrome occurs secondary to a flexion-compression injury. There is loss of neurological function of the anterior two-thirds of the spinal cord, namely the spinothalamic (pain, temperature) and corticospinal (motor) tracts. There is greater motor loss in the legs than the arms. The anterior cord syndrome has the worst prognosis of all spinal cord lesions.

Central cord syndrome is the most common spinal cord lesion. It occurs in older people with cervical spondylosis who sustain a hyperextension injury. There is a flaccid weakness of the arms, but motor and sensory fibres to the lower limb are comparatively preserved as these are located more peripherally in the spinal cord. Central cord lesions have a fair prognosis.

Hyperextension injuries can result in loss of dorsal column function (*posterior cord syndrome*). These injuries are very rare and the motor and sensory function is preserved. Gait is impaired due to impaired proprioception. The prognosis of posterior cord lesions is good.

37. TUMOUR MARKERS (2)

D – CEA

This man presents with a change in bowel habit, tenesmus and fatigue – symptoms typical of colorectal cancer. Carcinoembryonic antigen (CEA) is a tumour antigen which is associated with colorectal cancer. It is not specific or sensitive enough to be used by itself to make a diagnosis but can be used as a screening tool and to monitor relapse following treatment. CA 15-3, CA 125 and CA 19-9 are all monoclonal antibodies. CA 15-3 is associated with breast cancer, CA 125 with ovarian cancer and CA 19-9 with pancreatic and hepatobiliary cancers. Prostate specific antigen (PSA) is used in the screening and monitoring of prostate cancer.

Tenesmus, from Greek, *tenein* = to strain or stretch.

For a list of tumour markers, see the question 'Tumour markers (1)'.

38. MANAGING TESTICULAR PAIN (2)

A – Analgesia and bed rest

The history in this scenario is suggestive of mumps orchitis. Mumps orchitis is most common in pre-pubescent boys and occurs in around 20%, 4–7 days after parotitis. Orchitis is unilateral in 70% of cases. Presentation is with testicular pain, scrotal oedema and general systemic symptoms, e.g. fever and malaise. The diagnosis can be made on the history and examination alone, although it is important to exclude torsion if the cause is unclear (even if the only means is by scrotal exploration). Treatment is supportive and comprises adequate analgesia, bed rest, local ice packs and scrotal support. An associated tense hydrocele (collection of fluid within the tunica vaginalis) may need to be drained. Mumps orchitis is complicated by testicular atrophy in at least 50% and bilateral involvement may result in infertility. There is controversy about the association of mumps orchitis with the development of testicular cancer. Other causes of viral orchitis include infectious mononucleosis and varicella. Bacterial orchitis is most common in older males. Causes include sexually transmitted infections (e.g. chlamydia) and urinary stasis (as occurs in benign prostatic hypertrophy). Bacterial orchitis usually also involves the epididymis – epididymo-orchitis. Treatment is with appropriate antibiotics (a urine sample and urethral swabs must be taken as indicated).

39. ANORECTAL DISEASE (2)

C – Pilonidal sinus

A pilonidal sinus is a sinus that contains a tuft of hair. It is typically found within the natal cleft and is associated with dark hair, hirsutism and obesity. Pilonidal sinuses are most common in men. They may also occur in the web spaces of the fingers of barbers and farmers. The sinuses can cause pain and inflammation, and can present acutely as an abscess. Small sinuses may only require antibiotics, whereas larger problematic sinuses can be drained or excised and laid open. If a superimposing abscess has formed this must be drained and left to heal by secondary intention.

Rectal prolapse presents with the sensation of something coming down the back passage on defaecation; in the initial stages it may reduce spontaneously or with manual pressure. *Proctalgia fugax* is the name used to describe intermittent short-lasting spasms of rectal pain, which is unrelated to defaecation and typically worse at night. Examination of the patient is normal. A *perianal haematoma* occurs acutely when straining at stool and is caused by the rupture of a vein beneath the anal skin. A bluish bulge will be seen on examination and evacuation of the haematoma may be required.

40. MANAGING ARTERIAL DISEASE (1)

C – Start aspirin and refer for urgent inpatient assessment

This patient has presented with a history of transient ischaemic attacks (TIAs), a focal neurological deficit of vascular origin that resolves completely within 24 hours. There is a risk of stroke of up to 15% a year following TIAs. Modifiable risk factors must be addressed (smoking, hypertension, diabetes) and low dose aspirin commenced. Carotid bruits are not a reliable indicator of the extent of internal carotid stenosis and so need to be formally investigated by Doppler studies. A stenosis of 70–99% is an indication for surgery in this case.

Any patient presenting with a TIA should be risk stratified using the ABCD2 score as follows:

A Age >65 (1 point)
B Blood pressure >140 systolic or >90 diastolic (1 point)
C Unilateral weakness (2 points), speech disturbance (1 point)
D Duration >60 minutes (2 points), 10–59 minutes (1 point)
E Diabetes (1 point)

Of a total score of 7, patients with a score of 4 or more require admission for inpatient assessment regarding suitability for carotid endarterectomy. Similarly, patients with two or more episodes of TIA in quick succession ('crescendo TIA') also require urgent assessment regardless of their ABCD2 score. The patient in this scenario has an ABCD2 score of 5, and has had two episodes in quick succession, so requires inpatient assessment and urgent carotid endarterectomy if suitable.

41. SHOULDER DISORDERS (2)

B – Proximal rupture of biceps tendon

The biceps muscle has two sites of origin at the shoulder (the long and short head) and inserts into the tuberosity of the radius. Rupture of the biceps most commonly occurs proximally, at the site of origin of the long head, and presents with acute pain and the sensation of a 'snap'. After this, the retracted muscle is seen as a bulge in the upper arm, most obvious on flexion of the elbow (the 'Popeye muscle'). Proximal rupture of the biceps is most commonly seen after middle age in those with degenerative changes in the biceps tendon. In the young it is most often associated with weight lifting. Treatment is largely conservative, unless the patient is young and active, as shoulder function is maintained by the short head of the biceps. Distal rupture of the biceps tendon is much rarer (5% of cases) and occurs following flexion against resistance. It presents with acute pain, swelling and bruising of the elbow. The tendon may be palpable in the antecubital fossa. Again it is most common after middle age. Unlike proximal ruptures, treatment is largely by surgical reattachment to prevent weakness in flexion and supination.

Rupture of the triceps tendon is rare, usually occurring where there is pre-existing weakening. Causes include a fall onto the outstretched arm and pushing weights. Pain is felt acutely at the tip of the elbow, especially on trying to extend the arm, and there will be marked swelling posteriorly. Treatment is largely conservative. The rotator cuff is a ring of muscles and tendons that provide stability to the shoulder girdle. It is made up of four muscles: supraspinatus, infraspinatus, subscapularis and teres minor. *Rotator cuff tears* typically occur in older patients following trauma and usually involve the supraspinatus tendon. The most common site of the tear is the 'critical zone' of the supraspinatus tendon, a relatively avascular region near its insertion. Patients present with shoulder tip pain and an inability to abduct the arm. There is localized tenderness at the lateral margin of the acromion. If the arm is abducted to above 90 degrees with assistance then the patient can sustain the abduction by action of the deltoid muscle (the 'abduction paradox'). If the arm is lowered below 90 degrees it suddenly drops (the 'drop arm' sign). *Acute calcific tendonitis* of the supraspinatus tendon usually occurs in younger women. Deposition of calcium hydroxyapatite crystals on the medial insertion of the supraspinatus tendon results in acute onset severe shoulder pain. The pain is worst on abduction above 120 degrees – this is different to the range of maximal pain in the impingement syndrome (see below). The pain worsens over a few hours and gradually subsides over a few days.

In the *impingement syndrome* (a.k.a. painful arc syndrome) there is pain on arm abduction between 60 and 120 degrees only. The pain is produced by mechanical nipping of a tender structure between the greater tuberosity of the humerus and the acromion process. The primary lesions that give rise to the painful arc syndrome are: incomplete tear of supraspinatus, chronic supraspinatus tendonitis, subacromial bursitis and a crack fracture of the greater tuberosity.

42. LOIN PAIN

E – Renal colic

Renal colic is a common presenting condition in the emergency department. There is a lifetime risk of 10% in men (it is three times less common in women) and usually presents between the ages of 20 and 40. Renal colic that presents in the very young or older population is usually the result of a metabolic abnormality. Risk factors for renal colic include a family history (doubles the risk), dehydration, structural renal tract abnormalities and the use of diuretics (particularly thiazides). Particular metabolic abnormalities include increased excretion of calcium, oxalate and uric acid. The presenting symptoms include sudden-onset pain in the loin/lumbar region which radiates anteriorly to the groin and genitalia, associated with irritative urinary symptoms (frequency, dysuria and haematuria). Nausea and vomiting often occur. Typically the patient moves around, unable to get comfortable. There may be no particular signs on examination. In uncomplicated renal colic the patient will be afebrile. Investigation must include a urine dipstick (85% have microscopic haematuria) and bloods for urea and electrolytes. Appropriate imaging includes a KUB (kidney, ureter, bladder) X-ray (up to 90% of calculi are visible), ultrasound scanning and an intravenous pyelogram (IVP). IVP used to be the investigation of choice, but due to the risk of anaphylaxis and contrast nephropathy, spiral CT scanning (CT-KUB) without contrast has now become the 'gold standard'. Treatment of renal colic depends on the size of the stone. Small calculi (<5 mm) pass spontaneously in 90%, medium stones (5–9 mm) in 50% and those greater than 1 cm usually require intervention. Options for stone removal include extracorporeal shock wave lithotripsy, percutaneous nephrolithotomy and ureteroscopy +/– stent insertion. The most severe complications of renal calculi occur secondary to obstruction, and include renal failure and sepsis. If there is evidence of either an infected or obstructed kidney it is a urological emergency and a cystoscopically placed retrograde ureteric stent or a percutaneous nephrostomy may be required. *Renal cell carcinoma* is the most common cancer affecting the kidneys (85%). It typically presents in the fifth decade, the classic triad being haematuria, flank pain and a mass (often late in the disease). The majority of cases are picked up incidentally or on 2-week wait referrals for haematuria.

Risk factors include smoking, a family history and von Hippel-Lindau syndrome. Treatment of localized disease is with a nephrectomy. The survival in localized disease is 85% at 5 years, decreasing to 10% with metastatic disease. *Pyelonephritis* is inflammation of the kidney caused by an ascending bacterial urinary tract infection. It is most common in young women. It presents with urinary frequency, dysuria, fever and rigors. There is often marked tenderness in the renal angle. Treatment is with antibiotics.

43. DYSPHAGIA (2)

B – Oesophageal carcinoma

A history of rapidly progressive dysphagia with weight loss in a patient of this age (60–80 years) suggests a diagnosis of oesophageal carcinoma. Oesophageal carcinomas are mostly of the squamous cell type and risk factors for development include male sex, smoking, achalasia, alcohol use, gastro-oesophageal reflux disease, Barrett's oesophagus, coeliac disease and Chinese ethnicity. Squamous cell carcinomas of the oesophagus occur most frequently in the mid-oesophagus and spread of tumours is to local structures, such as the trachea and recurrent laryngeal nerve (blood metastases occur late). Adenocarcinomas of the oesophagus are much rarer and arise in the lower third of the oesophagus. They are associated with long-standing gastrooesophageal reflux and the development of Barrett's oesophagus (gastric/intestinal metaplasia of the distal oesophagus). The diagnosis of oesophageal carcinoma is by endoscopy and biopsy, with a CT scan performed later to stage the disease. A barium swallow will show an irregular filling defect.

Treatment is dependent on the size and spread of the tumour. A curative option is oesophagectomy with re-anastomosis of the stomach to the upper oesophagus. Patients with unresectable tumours may be given palliative stenting or radiotherapy to improve dysphagia. Oesophageal tumours have a poor prognosis.

Oesophageal candidiasis results from infection of the oesophagus by *Candida albicans.* It commonly arises in the setting of immunosuppression (e.g. acquired immunodeficiency syndrome, diabetes or steroid use) or in those who have recently used antibiotics. Patients often complain of dysphagia, odynophagia and a hoarse voice. Raised white plaques which can be removed by the endoscope are seen on endoscopy. Treatment is with antifungals such as fluconazole. *Oesophageal spasm* is a disorder of oesophageal motility. It is subdivided into a 'diffuse type', where contractions are uncoordinated (causing dysphagia and regurgitation), and a 'nutcracker type', where contractions are coordinated but occur at a higher than normal amplitude (causing odynophagia). Oesophageal spasm is most common in elderly women. Diagnosis is by barium swallow and manometry. *Oesophageal webs* are thin membranes of tissue which form within the oesophagus (some may be congenital) and cause dysphagia (worse with solids) and reflux. They are most common in Caucasian women. The Plummer–Vinson (or Paterson–Brown-Kelly) syndrome describes the presence of an oesophageal web with chronic iron deficiency anaemia. It is a risk factor for the development of oesophageal carcinoma. *Oesophageal strictures* may be benign or malignant. Causes include intraluminal pathology (malignancy, fibrosis secondary to long-standing GORD), extra-luminal pathology (compressive tumours of the bronchus) and abnormalities in peristalsis (oesophageal spasm).

Norman Rupert Barrett, British surgeon (1903–1979).

44. PAEDIATRIC ORTHOPAEDICS (2)

B – Perthes disease

Perthes disease (or Legg-Calvé-Perthes disease) describes idiopathic avascular necrosis of the femoral head, which is followed by revascularization and reossification over a period of 2–3 years. It usually occurs between the ages of 5 and 10 and is five times more common in boys. In 10% of patients the condition is bilateral. Presentation is insidious with hip pain (which may be referred to the groin or knee) and a limp. Examination may reveal a reduced range of movements in all directions of the hip joint, secondary to irritation of the capsule, although internal rotation and abduction are usually more affected. There may be a fixed flexion deformity of the opposite leg (to compensate for shortening of the affected leg) and there may be some muscle wasting on the affected side. X-ray will show a collapsed, irregular, sclerotic femoral head (secondary to osteopenia of surrounding bone) with an increased joint space. MRI may be more sensitive in detecting changes early on in the condition. Treatment depends upon the extent of disease and the amount of femoral head involved. Mild disease may be treated conservatively with bed rest, analgesia and repeat imaging to monitor progress. More severe disease may be treated by abduction bracing/splinting or by femoral osteotomy. The prognosis is worse the older the child, in girls and if more than half the femoral head is affected. Complications include early osteoarthritis and coxa magna (overgrowth of the femoral head).

Georg Clemens Perthes, German surgeon (1869–1927).

45. FOOT DISORDERS (2)

E – March fracture

March fractures are undisplaced hairline fractures caused by repetitive stress, e.g. marching or running. They commonly occur near the neck of the second or third metatarsal. X-ray may be normal in a majority of cases, although a periosteal reaction of callus formation may be seen.

Treatment is with analgesia and the pain resolves after a few weeks when fracture union occurs.

A *Jones fracture* is a fracture of the proximal end of the fifth metatarsal. A *Lisfranc fracture* is a fracture dislocation of the midfoot, disrupting the joint between the second to fourth metatarsals and the underlying cuneiforms. *Hallux rigidus* is the name given to osteoarthritis of the first metatarsophalangeal joint. It presents with localized pain, which then radiates over the foot, and stiffness of the big toe. It is more common in active individuals.

46. ULCERS (2)

D – Marjolin ulcer

A Marjolin ulcer is an aggressive but slow-growing squamous cell carcinoma that arises within an area of previously traumatized skin (e.g. burns, scars, chronic wounds). Lesions are typically raised, ulcerated and painless, and invade locally. Diagnosis is made on biopsy and treatment is by wide local excision.

Hypertrophic and keloid scars occur when there is an overgrowth of fibrous tissue within a healing scar. Hypertrophic scars present as raised lesions which occur within the boundary of the original scar whereas keloid scars extend beyond the original scar. Symptoms include pain and pruritus, and keloid scars in particular may cause significant cosmetic concern to the patient. If scarring occurs across joints, contractures may result in loss of joint function. Keloid and hypertrophic scarring is most common in those of Afro-Caribbean origin and occurs most commonly on the face, trunk and back. Hypertrophic scars have the ability to spontaneously regress.

An ulcer may be defined as a breach in the skin or mucous membrane. Complications of ulcers in general include infection (as occurs in venous ulcers), perforation (as occurs in peptic ulcers) and malignant transformation (as above).

Jean Nicholas Marjolin, French surgeon (1780–1850).

47. THE SWOLLEN LIMB (2)

A – Filariasis

Filariasis is a cause of secondary lymphoedema. Filariasis (a.k.a. elephantiasis) is characterized by thickening of the skin and subcutaneous tissues, often of the legs and genitals. It is caused by infection and obstruction of lymph vessels by the parasite *Wuchereria bancrofti* in tropical countries. The infection is transmitted by mosquito bites.

Elephantiasis, from the Greek *elephantas* = elephant; describing the appearance of the limbs in the affected patient.

48. INVESTIGATING DYSPHAGIA (2)

A – 24-hour lower oesophageal pH

This patient has presented with symptoms of gastro-oesophageal reflux disease (GORD). GORD arises because of an abnormally low resting tone of the lower oesophageal sphincter, allowing the reflux of gastric contents back into the oesophagus. Symptoms include retrosternal and epigastric burning pain, waterbrash and nocturnal cough. Symptoms are exacerbated by eating, bending forwards and lying down. GORD is associated with hiatus hernias, smoking, pregnancy and being overweight. Long-standing GORD can lead to oesophagitis, stricture formation, iron deficiency anaemia and adenocarcinoma of the oesophagus.

The diagnosis of reflux can be made by measuring the lower oesophageal pH. A pH probe is inserted into the lower oesophagus and left for 24 hours – if the pH is less than 4 for more than 4 hours then oesophageal reflux is confirmed. Management of reflux can be conservative (weight loss, diet changes, antacids), medical or surgical. Drugs used to manage GORD include proton pump inhibitors such as omeprazole. Surgical repair of medically resistant reflux is with Nissen's fundoplication, where the fundus of the stomach is wrapped around the lower oesophagus. A barium swallow provides images of the anatomy and function of the upper GI tract, a chest X-ray may occasionally reveal a hiatus hernia (air–fluid level behind the heart), endoscopy allows direct visualization of the upper GI tract, and manometry assesses the pressures within the oesophagus.

Rudolph Nissen, German surgeon (1896–1981).

49. UPPER LIMB NERVE LESIONS (1)

B – Wasting of the hand, except the thenar eminence, and clawing of the ring and little fingers

The ulnar nerve is susceptible to damage in elbow fractures as it runs behind the medial epicondyle. An ulnar nerve lesion at the elbow would result in: wasting of the flexor carpi ulnaris and flexor digitorum, wasting of the small muscles of the hand *except* the thenar eminence and lateral two lumbricals (supplied by the median nerve), and clawing of the ring and little fingers. There will be an inability to abduct and adduct the fingers (caused by paralysis of the interossei), an inability to adduct the thumb (as suggested by Froment sign where one cannot hold a piece of paper in a pinching grip between thumb and index finger), an inability to abduct the little finger (paralysis of hypothenar muscles), and loss of sensation over the ulnar one and a half fingers. With more distal ulnar lesions, the clawing is more marked (the ulnar paradox). This is because the flexor digitorum profundus, which is supplied by the proximal ulnar nerve, is intact in distal lesions, resulting in more flexion of the interphalangeal joints and an exacerbated flexion deformity. With ulnar lesions at the wrist, sensation is not affected due to sparing of the dorsal cutaneous branch. Wrist drop with lack of sensation over the anatomical snuff box is seen in radial nerve injuries, while wasting of the thenar eminence and inability to abduct the thumb occur in median nerve injuries.

50. ABDOMINAL PAIN (6)

D – Torsion of the ovary

Torsion of the ovary is an unusual but important cause of an acute abdomen in women. It commonly occurs in young women (70% are under the age of 30) and up to 20% occur during pregnancy. In the majority of cases torsion is associated with an abnormally enlarged ovary (which may be benign or malignant). Other associations include anatomical abnormalities, e.g. abnormally long fallopian tubes, and fertility treatment where excessive cyst stimulation causes generalized enlargement of the ovary. Ovarian torsion more frequently occurs on the right side and there may be a history of previous episodes of pain caused by intermittent twisting. Left untreated, a torted ovary will undergo necrosis causing peritonitis (with a risk of reduced future fertility). Diagnosis is largely one of exclusion (i.e. excluding appendicitis and ectopic pregnancy). Both ultrasound and CT scanning are useful imaging techniques; however laparoscopy will allow diagnosis and treatment in one procedure. If there are no signs of vascular compromise, peritonitis or malignancy within the ovary, the ovary may be 'untwisted' and fixed (oophoropexy). Otherwise a salpingo-oophorectomy is performed.

Practice Papers 3: Questions

1. UPPER LIMB NERVE LESIONS (2)

A 36-year-old man presents to the emergency department following a road traffic collision. He has fractured his right tibia and also complains of pain in his neck. On examination, he is unable to lift his right arm, which is medially rotated and extended at the elbow. There is a loss of sensation on the lateral side of the right arm and forearm.

Which nerve has most likely been affected?

A. Lower brachial plexus
B. Median nerve
C. Radial nerve
D. Ulnar nerve
E. Upper brachial plexus

2. ABDOMINAL INCISIONS (2)

A 19-year-old man is brought into the emergency department following a gunshot wound to the abdomen. Despite resuscitation he remains haemodynamically unstable. The decision is made to take him to theatre for exploration.

Which of the following surgical incisions would be most appropriate?

A. Battle incision
B. Median thoracotomy
C. Midline laparotomy
D. Pfannenstiel incision
E. Thoraco-abdominal incision

3. SHOCK (3)

A 34-year-old man has presented to the emergency department following a large haematemesis. On examination, the patient appears agitated. His pulse is 120/min, blood pressure 122/84 mmHg and respiratory rate 22/ min.

How would you classify the patient's current condition?

A. Class I haemorrhagic shock
B. Class II haemorrhagic shock

C. Class III haemorrhagic shock
D. Class IV haemorrhagic shock
E. Class V haemorrhagic shock

4. ULCERS (3)

A 52-year-old woman attends the GP practice having noticed a crater-like lesion on the sole of her right foot. She has a history of type 2 diabetes mellitus and hypertension. On examination, the lesion is painless.
What is the most likely diagnosis?

A. Diabetic dermopathy
B. Necrobiosis lipoidica
C. Neuropathic ulcer
D. Pyoderma gangrenosum
E. Vitiligo

5. ABDOMINAL PAIN (7)

A 54-year-old man presents with a 2-day history of upper abdominal and shoulder tip pain on the right side. He also complains of difficulty breathing and episodes of fever and sweats. He underwent a laparotomy 2 weeks ago following a perforated appendix.
What is the most likely diagnosis?

A. Appendix abscess
B. Cholecystitis
C. Diverticular abscess
D. Polycystic liver disease
E. Subphrenic abscess

6. GLASGOW COMA SCORE (1)

An 18-year-old has been physically assaulted outside a bar. On arrival at the emergency department she appears drowsy and there is gross swelling to the right side of her face. On examination, she is making groaning sounds but is not verbally interactive. She is unable to obey commands but withdraws to pain and opens her eyes only to painful stimulus.
What is her Glasgow coma score?

A. 3
B. 6
C. 8
D. 10
E. 13

7. ABDOMINAL PAIN (8)

A 24-year-old man, who has been suffering from intermittent fresh bleeding per rectum, presents to the emergency department with a 6-hour history of right-sided abdominal pain, fevers and nausea. On examination, he has tenderness and guarding in the right iliac fossa. His temperature is 38.2°C.

What is the most likely diagnosis?

A. Appendicitis
B. Haemorrhoids
C. Meckel diverticulitis
D. Renal colic
E. *Shigella* infection

8. DYSPHAGIA (3)

A 72-year-old man presents with difficulty swallowing and regurgitation of food. He has also had several chest infections over the last few months. On examination, you see a soft swelling in the anterior triangle of the neck. On palpation, the swelling makes a gurgling sound.

What is the most likely cause of his dysphagia?

A. Carotid artery aneurysm
B. Enlarged lymph node
C. Laryngocoele
D. Pharyngeal pouch
E. Thyroglossal cyst

9. FLUID THERAPY (2)

A 22-year-old man is brought in following a road traffic collision. He is suspected to have intra-abdominal injuries and there is bruising over his trunk. On arrival, he has a pulse rate of 140/min and his systolic blood pressure is 80 mmHg.

Which of the following fluids would raise the patient's blood pressure most rapidly?

A. 5% dextrose
B. Fresh frozen plasma
C. Packed red cells
D. Mannitol
E. Normal saline

10. MANAGING ANORECTAL DISEASE (3)

A 36-year-old man presents to the surgical outpatient clinic with a 3-week history of soiled underwear. He is known to have Crohn disease. On examination, an opening is seen at the posterior margin of the anus which is discharging faeculent material. Subsequent imaging demonstrates an anal fistula that tracks through the puborectalis muscle.

What would be the most appropriate management of this condition?

A. Diltiazem ointment
B. Excision of the fistula

C. Laying open of the fistula tract

D. Lord procedure

E. Seton insertion

11. ANATOMY OF HERNIAS (1)

Which term best fits the description of the hernia given below?

This hernia arises from a triangle bounded by the external oblique muscle, the latissimus dorsi and the iliac crest below.

A. Amyand

B. Littre

C. Lumbar

D. Obturator

E. Sciatic

12. TESTICULAR DISEASE

A 27-year-old man presents to the GP practice having noticed a painless swelling of his right testicle. He is otherwise well. On examination, the testis is enlarged, firm and has a nodular texture.

What is the most likely diagnosis?

A. Epididymal cyst

B. Gumma

C. Haematocele

D. Orchitis

E. Testicular cancer

13. BREAST DISEASE (3)

A 58-year-old woman presents with itchy, dry skin around the left areola. On examination, the skin is dry and cracked, and there appears to be a 1 cm nodule underlying the affected area.

What is the most likely diagnosis?

A. Atopic dermatitis

B. Fibrocystic disease

C. Mondor disease

D. Paget disease

E. Peau d'orange

14. INVESTIGATING DYSPHAGIA (3)

A 7-year-old boy is brought to the emergency department by his father, having told him that he had swallowed a five pence coin earlier that day. The child has not experienced any symptoms and on examination is well.

Which of the following investigations would you perform in the first instance?

A. Barium swallow
B. Laryngoscopy
C. Neck, chest and abdominal X-rays
D. No investigation required
E. Upper gastrointestinal endoscopy

15. ENDOCRINE DISEASE (3)

A 37-year-old man presents to the GP with a 2-month history of thirst and frequency of urination. He has no significant past medical history and examination is unremarkable. Routine bloods demonstrate the following: random glucose 5.6 mmol/L, sodium 142 mmol/L and potassium 2.9 mmol/L.

What is the most likely diagnosis?

A. Addison disease
B. Congenital adrenal hyperplasia
C. Conn syndrome
D. Multiple endocrine neoplasia
E. Phaeochromocytoma

16. INVESTIGATING GI BLEEDING

A 74-year-old woman presents to the emergency department complaining of dizziness and tiredness. On direct questioning she tells you she has recently been having black stools. She is currently awaiting a total hip replacement for arthritis.

Which of the following would be most useful in establishing the primary cause of her symptoms?

A. Barium meal
B. Coagulation screen
C. Faecal occult blood
D. Full blood count
E. Oesophagogastroduodenoscopy

17. SKIN LESIONS (3)

A 42-year-old woman presents to her GP with a new rash on her left hand. She has a history of diabetes mellitus. On examination, the lesion is on the dorsal hand and is made up of reddish bumps arranged in a ring. She is otherwise well.

What is the most likely diagnosis?

A. Dercum disease
B. Granuloma annulare
C. Lipoma
D. Pyogenic granuloma
E. Seborrhoeic keratosis

18. INVESTIGATING ENDOCRINE DISEASE (3)

A 6-year-old girl is referred by her GP to the paediatric clinic with preco-cious puberty. On examination, she is found to have clitoromegaly and some pubic hair. She is on the 98th centile for height and weight.

Which of the following will be most helpful in determining the under-lying diagnosis?

A. 17-hydroxyprogesterone levels
B. 24-hour urinary vanillylmandelic acid
C. 24-hour urinary 5-hydroxyindole acetic acid
D. Serum calcitonin
E. Short synacthen test

19. MANAGING SKIN CONDITIONS (1)

A 6-year-old girl is brought to the emergency department with multiple crusted lesions on her face which have spread over the last two days. They are very itchy and often bleed. She is otherwise well.

Which of the following is the most appropriate course of management?

A. Analgesia
B. Intravenous antibiotics
C. Oral antibiotics
D. Surgical excision
E. Reassurance

20. NECK LUMPS (3)

A 42-year-old man presents to the GP with a slowly enlarging mass in the left side of his neck which has been present for 3 months. On examina-tion, the mass is 2 cm in diameter, non-tender, pulsatile and can be moved from side to side, but not up or down.

What is the most likely diagnosis?

A. Branchial cyst
B. Cervical rib
C. Chemodectoma
D. Pleomorphic adenoma
E. Virchow node

21. EPISTAXIS

A 23-year-old man presents to the emergency department with a nose bleed. He tells you this has been a recent recurrent problem and that his father was the same. On examination, you note that he has multiple dilated blood vessels around the nose and mouth.

Which of the following is the most likely cause of his epistaxis?

A. Haemophilia B
B. Hypertension

C. Osler-Weber-Rendu syndrome
D. Septal polyps
E. Sturge-Weber syndrome

22. KNEE CONDITIONS (1)

A 33-year-old man presents to the emergency department with an acutely painful swollen right knee. On examination, he has a swollen, red hot knee with minimal range of movement. Aspiration of the joint shows turbulent fluid with a raised neutrophil count and no crystals.

What is the most likely diagnosis?

A. Gout
B. Pseudogout
C. Reiter's syndrome
D. Rheumatoid arthritis
E. Septic arthritis

23. CHEST TRAUMA (3)

A 22-year-old man is brought into the resuscitation room with multiple stab wounds to the chest. On arrival he is tachycardic, hypotensive and has engorged jugular veins. His heart sounds are barely audible on auscultation.

Which of the following is the most likely cause of his symptoms?

A. Cardiac tamponade
B. Cardiogenic shock
C. Haemothorax
D. Haemorrhagic shock
E. Tension pneumothorax

24. HERNIAS (3)

A 42-year-old woman presents with an upper midline mass that has been present for over a year. She has a history of a partial gastrectomy for a perforated ulcer. On examination, the mass is 5 cm in size, soft, non-tender and reducible.

Which of the following is the most likely diagnosis?

A. Direct inguinal hernia
B. Epigastric hernia
C. Hiatus hernia
D. Incisional hernia
E. Paraumbilical hernia

25. CERVICAL SPINE MANAGEMENT

An 18-year-old boy is brought into the emergency department having fallen down a flight of stairs outside his flat. His cervical spine is immobilized by the attending paramedics. The patient is saying he does not have neck pain and wants the collar removed.

In which of the following circumstances is it appropriate to remove the collar?

A. He has been drinking alcohol
B. He has lost consciousness for only 5 minutes
C. He has no cervical spine tenderness
D. He is in shock with a splenic injury which requires a laparotomy
E. He has no peripheral neurological signs

26. PAEDIATRIC ORTHOPAEDICS (3)

An 18-month-old girl has been referred to the orthopaedic outpatient clinic. Her mother has noticed that she is walking with an increasing limp on the left side. The girl denies any pain. A pelvic X-ray shows a vertically orientated acetabular roof and poorly developed femoral head.

What is the most likely diagnosis?

A. Developmental dysplasia of the hip
B. Genu valgum
C. Genu varum
D. Perthes disease
E. Slipped upper femoral epiphysis

27. JAUNDICE (3)

A 27-year-old man presents to the GP with a sore throat and fevers. On examination, you notice that he is jaundiced and the tonsils are inflamed. On direct questioning the patient tells you that he has noticed this discolouration of his skin before, particularly when run down or after drinking alcohol. His blood tests are all normal except for a mildly raised bilirubin.

What is the most likely diagnosis?

A. Alcoholic hepatitis
B. Gallstones
C. Gilbert syndrome
D. Type 1 Crigler-Najjar syndrome
E. Viral hepatitis

28. MANAGING UROLOGICAL DISEASE (1)

You are called to see a 62-year-old man on the ward who was admitted earlier in the day with frank haematuria with the passage of clots. He is now complaining of lower abdominal pain and an inability to pass urine. On examination the bladder is distended.

Which of the following would you perform in the first instance?

A. Catheterization using a Foley catheter
B. Catheterization using a three-way catheter

C. Cystoscopy
D. Suprapubic catheterization
E. Ultrasound of the bladder

29. GROIN LUMPS (3)

A 40-year-old man is being investigated for an enlarging painless lump in the right testicle. Blood results show a significantly raised alpha fetoprotein and a normal beta-hCG.

Which of the following testicular tumours is most likely to be the cause of his symptoms?

A. Choriocarcinoma
B. Leydig cell tumour
C. Seminoma
D. Testicular lymphoma
E. Yolk sac carcinoma

30. MANAGING BILIARY TRACT DISEASE

A 38-year-old woman who has a history of intermittent right upper quadrant pain associated with eating, attends the emergency department with a 3-day history of severe, unremitting abdominal pain and jaundice. A bedside ultrasound scan shows a 1 cm stone in her common bile duct.

Which of the following would be most suitable management?

A. Cholecystectomy
B. ERCP
C. Fragmentation of the stone
D. Laparotomy
E. MRCP

31. INVESTIGATING ABDOMINAL PAIN (3)

A 65-year-old woman with a past medical history of hypertension and stable angina presents to the GP practice complaining of episodes of severe central abdominal pain. They occur around half an hour after meals and can last up to an hour. She is becoming reluctant to eat because of the pain and as a result she has lost nearly a stone in weight over the past 2 months. Examination is unremarkable.

Which of these investigations would be the most informative?

A. Barium follow through
B. CT scan
C. Colonoscopy
D. Exercise tolerance test
E. Mesenteric angiography

32. PENILE CONDITIONS (1)

A 27-year-old man who has just returned from a holiday in Asia presents to the GP surgery having noticed a painless hard ulcer over the penile glans. He is otherwise well. On examination, the patient has generalized painless lymphadenopathy.

Which of the following is the most likely cause of his symptoms?

A. *Escherichia coli*
B. *Haemophilus ducreyi*
C. Herpes simplex virus
D. Human papilloma virus
E. *Treponema pallidum*

33. BONE PAIN (1)

A 69-year-old man presents with a 6-week history of lower back and right hip pain. An X-ray of the hip shows an osteosclerotic lesion in the proximal femur. On direct questioning he tells you he has been having problems passing urine over the past few months.

Which of the following is the most likely cause of his symptoms?

A. Benign prostatic hypertrophy
B. Paget disease
C. Prostatic carcinoma
D. Prostatitis
E. Testicular carcinoma

34. INVESTIGATING VASCULAR DISEASE (1)

A 65-year-old man presents to the vascular outpatient clinic with a history of severe cramping pains in the right calf on walking. The pain has been so severe that he has had to stop his activities. Over the last few months he has also had pain at rest, particularly at night, which is relieved on hanging his leg off the bed. Examination of the right leg shows it is cool and there is difficulty palpating the pulses. There are no gangrenous changes or ulcers.

Which of the following ankle brachial pressure index results would you expect?

A. 0.1
B. 0.3
C. 0.7
D. 1.0
E. 1.4

35. ABDOMINAL PAIN (9)

A 34-year-old man presents to the emergency department with a 6-hour history of abdominal pain and vomiting. On examination, the abdomen is distended and tympanic. He tells you that for the last 6 months he has been having episodes of cramping right-sided abdominal pain with intermittent episodes of blood in his stools.

Which of the following complications has resulted in his presentation today?

A. Abscess formation
B. Fistula formation
C. Primary sclerosing cholangitis
D. Stricture formation
E. Toxic megacolon

36. HEPATOMEGALY (3)

A 27-year-old man presents with fevers and right lower abdominal pain following a 1-week history of bloody diarrhoea. He has recently returned from holiday in the Maldives, but has previously been fit and well. On examination, he has a tender palpable liver.

Which of the following is the most likely cause of his symptoms?

A. Acute cholecystitis
B. Amoebic liver abscess
C. Fitz-Hugh–Curtis syndrome
D. Polycystic liver
E. Pyogenic liver abscess

37. MANAGEMENT OF ARTERIAL DISEASE (2)

A 72-year-old man presents to the emergency department with a 3-hour history of a painful, cold right leg. He has a past medical history of atrial fibrillation. On examination, the right leg is cold and tender. The pedal pulses on the right are not palpable.

What would be the most appropriate initial management?

A. Amputation
B. Aorto-bifemoral bypass graft
C. Conservative management
D. Embolectomy
E. Fasciotomy

38. HAND DISORDERS (1)

A 33-year-old man presents to the emergency department having hit the end of his finger with a hammer while at work. He is now unable to lift the end of his finger. On examination, the index finger is flexed at the distal interphalangeal joint.

Which of the following is the most likely diagnosis?

A. Boutonniere deformity
B. Duck bill deformity

C. Mallet finger
D. Swan neck deformity
E. Trigger finger

39. MANAGING ANORECTAL DISEASE (1)

A 27-year-old man with a long history of constipation presents with a history of severe pain on defaecation and bright red blood on the tissue paper. On examination, you see a skin tag at the anal verge. Per rectum examination is not possible due to severe pain.

Which of the following treatments would you suggest?

A. Analgesic suppositories
B. Excision of skin tag
C. Haemorrhoidectomy
D. Incision and drainage
E. Topical GTN ointment

40. BACK PAIN (1)

A 34-year-old builder comes to see you in the GP practice complaining of a 3-week history of lower back ache. The pain is worst at the end of the day and partially relieved by lying down. He has no other associated symptoms of note. Examination is unremarkable.

What would be the most suitable management option in the first instance?

A. Blood tests for ESR and bone profile
B. Lumbar X-ray
C. Refer for MRI of the spine
D. Simple analgesia and bed rest
E. Simple analgesia and gentle mobilization

41. MANAGING ABDOMINAL PAIN (3)

A 25-year-old woman has been investigated with lower gastrointestinal endoscopy and biopsy following complaints of frequent bloody diarrhoea which is still continuing. The results show diffuse superficial inflammation with ulceration in the rectum only.

Which of the following treatment options would be most suitable in the first instance?

A. Azathioprine
B. Colectomy
C. Mesalazine
D. Prednisolone
E. Surveillance colonoscopy

42. SPINAL CORD LESIONS (3)

A 67-year-old woman was gardening at home when she developed sudden-onset lower back pain. She found it difficult to get back into the house before she called an ambulance. She now has pain in both her legs and is unable to pass urine. On examination, there is reduced sensation around the perineum.

What is the most likely diagnosis?

A. Anterior cord syndrome
B. Brown-Séquard syndrome
C. Cauda equina syndrome
D. Posterior cord syndrome
E. Syringomyelia

43. MANAGING BREAST CANCER

A 46-year-old pre-menopausal woman has a 5 cm lump over her right breast which has been confirmed to be an invasive tumour. She is otherwise fit and well.

Which is the next most appropriate course of action?

A. Mastectomy
B. Radiotherapy
C. Tamoxifen
D. Trastuzumab
E. Wide local excision

44. FOOT DISORDERS (3)

A 38-year-old man presents to the emergency department. He says that while playing football he felt like he had been kicked in the back of the ankle and fell to the floor. He now has severe pain in his ankle on weight bearing.

Which of the following is the most likely cause of his problem?

A. Achilles tendonitis
B. Achilles tendon rupture
C. Calcaneal fracture
D. Calcaneal spur
E. Posterior cruciate ligament rupture

45. THYROID DISEASE (3)

A 36-year-old woman presents to the GP with a 2-month history of tremors. This is interfering with her work as a typist and the worry has caused her to lose over a stone in weight over the last few weeks. On examination, the thyroid appears normal although a bruit can be heard overlying it.

What is the most likely diagnosis?

A. De Quervain thyroiditis
B. Graves disease
C. Thyroid adenoma
D. Thyroid storm
E. Toxic multinodular goitre

46. SALTER–HARRIS FRACTURES

A 6-year-old boy has a fall onto his outstretched hand. On examination, he is tender over the distal radius. An X-ray confirms a fracture through the distal radius growth plate which includes a metaphyseal and epiphyseal fragment.

What classification is most suitable for this fracture?

A. Salter–Harris I
B. Salter–Harris II
C. Salter–Harris III
D. Salter–Harris IV
E. Salter–Harris V

47. PAEDIATRIC SURGICAL MANAGEMENT (3)

A 5-year-old boy is brought into the resuscitation room with acute difficulty breathing. His mother tells you that he has been complaining of a sore throat for the past 2 days. On arrival he is febrile, tachypnoeic, sitting upright and drooling at the mouth. There is no ENT on call in the hospital.

Which of the following would you do as a priority?

A. Assess the back of the throat using a tongue depressor
B. Attempt to perform a fibre-optic laryngoscopy
C. Contact the anaesthetist on call and ask them to attend urgently
D. Give oral antibiotics
E. Request an urgent lateral radiograph of the neck

48. BURNS (1)

A 60-year-old woman was involved in a house fire and is brought to the emergency department. She has partial thickness burns over the whole of her left arm and superficial burns covering her back.

Estimate the percentage burn she has sustained.

A. 9%
B. 18%
C. 20%
D. 27%
E. 36%

49. LOWER LIMB NERVE LESIONS (3)

A 46-year-old woman has been involved in a road traffic collision. Her right knee hit the dashboard of the car. On arrival at the emergency department she is unable to flex her toes on the right side. Examination reveals an absence of the ankle jerk and loss of sensation over the sole of the right foot.

Which of the following nerves is most likely to have been affected?

A. Femoral nerve
B. Obturator nerve
C. Sciatic nerve
D. Sural nerve
E. Tibial nerve

50. PAEDIATRIC SURGERY (3)

An 8-year-old boy is brought into the emergency department by his father with a 1-day history of fever, right-sided abdominal pain and diarrhoea. He has no past medical history of note, but has recently recovered from a cold. On examination, he has a temperature of 39°C and is tender, but not guarding, in the right iliac fossa.

What is the most likely diagnosis?

A. Appendicitis
B. Crohn disease
C. Coeliac disease
D. Gastroenteritis
E. Mesenteric adenitis

Practice Paper 3: Answers

1. UPPER LIMB NERVE LESIONS (2)

E – Upper brachial plexus

Upper brachial plexus injuries, also known as Erb's palsy, involve the C5 and C6 nerve roots (the brachial plexus is made up of the roots C5 to T1). They are commonly caused by traction injuries, e.g. motorcycle accidents or birth injuries (due to pulling on the baby's arm). There is flaccid paralysis of the arm abductors, lateral rotators of the shoulder and supinators, so the affected arm hangs limp, is medially rotated, extended at the elbow and pronated with the hand pointing backwards – the waiter's tip position. Paralysis is accompanied by loss of sensation over the lateral arm and forearm.

Lower brachial plexus injuries, also known as Klumpke's palsy, involve the C8 and T1 nerve roots. They are often caused by breech birth injuries (when the baby's arm remains above its head) and motorcycle accidents. Patients present with a claw hand in all digits (from paralysis of the intrinsic muscles of the hand) and sensory loss along the ulnar border of the forearm and hand.

Wilhelm Heinrich Erb, German neurologist (1840–1921).

Augusta Marie Dejerine-Klumpke, French neurologist (1859–1927).

2. ABDOMINAL INCISIONS (2)

C – Midline laparotomy

The site of blood loss in this patient is unknown, so an incision that is quick to perform and allows easy access to the gut is required, and a midline laparotomy is the most suitable. A midline incision is made through the linea alba – a relatively avascular incision that can be made, extended and closed easily. However, midline incisions cross Langer's lines and thus are cosmetically poor.

Thoraco-abdominal incisions allow access to the lower thorax and upper abdomen by making a communication between the pleural and peritoneal cavities. A right-sided incision can be used in a hepatic resection and left-sided in resection of the lower oesophagus. Most laparotomy incisions can be extended into the chest if required. A thoracotomy is an incision made through the chest, performed in order to gain access to the thoracic organs. The Pfannenstiel incision is a transverse one made 5 cm above the pubic symphysis and around 10–12 cm across in the midline. It is used commonly by gynaecologists (for Caesarean sections and ovarian operations) and urologists (for access to the bladder and prostate). The Pfannenstiel incision offers excellent cosmetic results. A Battle incision was a vertical incision made just medial to the lateral border of the abdominal rectus muscle. It was previously used for appendicitis but is not recommended any more as it damages nerves entering the rectus sheath and carries a high risk of incisional hernia.

Hans Hermann Johannes Pfannenstiel, German gynaecologist (1862–1909).

William Henry Battle, English surgeon (1855–1936).

3. SHOCK (3)

B – Class II haemorrhagic shock

Shock is a life-threatening condition in which there is insufficient tissue perfusion, leading to inadequate oxygenation of organs which, if left untreated, will result in multi-organ failure and death. The causes of shock may be broadly classified according to their aetiology into hypovolaemic, cardiogenic, anaphylactic, septic and neurogenic.

Hypovolaemic shock results from rapid fluid loss resulting in an insufficient circulating volume. Causes include massive blood loss (haemorrhagic shock), burns and diarrhoea. Haemorrhagic shock may be classified further according to the percentage of blood loss as follows:

	Class 1	Class II	Class III	Class IV
Fluid loss	<15% <750 mL	15–30% 750–1500 mL	30–40% 1500–2000 mL	>40% >2000 mL
Heart rate (bpm)	<100	100–120	120–140	>140
Blood pressure	Normal	Normal, reduced pulse pressure	Low	Very low
Respiratory rate (breaths/min)	Normal (<20)	Slightly raised (20–30)	Tachypnoeic (30–40)	Very tachypnoeic (>40)
Urine output (mL/h)	>30	20–30	10–20	<10
Mental status	Alert	Anxious	Drowsy	Confused/ unconscious

The mainstay of managing haemorrhagic shock is fluid/blood replacement while attempting to prevent further loss. The above markers can also be used to monitor the patient's response. Note that blood pressure is not a sensitive indicator of shock, so do not wait for it to fall – by the time this happens the patient may have lost at least 30% of their circulating blood volume.

4. ULCERS (3)

C – Neuropathic ulcer

Neuropathic ulcers occur when there is a loss of protective sensation in the lower limbs resulting in unnoticed damage to the feet with the development of painless ulcers. This can follow trivial trauma. Ulcers typically occur over weight-bearing surfaces, such as the metatarsal heads. The typical sensory loss in diabetes is in a 'glove and stocking' distribution (distal arms and legs). It is therefore important that diabetics receive regular foot check-ups as part of their on-going management.

Necrobiosis lipoidica (necrobiosis lipoidica diabeticorum) begins as small, raised, red areas which gradually grow to become large, flat, waxy lesions that are reddish-brown or yellow in colour. They usually occur on the shins. Although most patients who develop necrobiosis lipoidica are diabetic, only 1% of diabetics have this condition.

Diabetic dermopathy (shin spots) are round areas of shiny, atrophic, pigmented skin that occur on the shins. They result from microvascular changes. They are largely asymptomatic but may occasionally itch or burn. The presence of more than four lesions is usually indicative of diabetes.

Vitiligo is a chronic skin condition characterized by irregular patches of depigmented skin, secondary to the destruction of melanocytes. Patches may occur anywhere on the body. It is in part an autoimmune condition and is associated with type 1 diabetes mellitus.

Pyoderma gangrenosum is a skin condition that is associated with inflammatory bowel disease, rheumatoid arthritis and myeloid blood dyscrasias (e.g. acute and chronic myeloid leukaemias). It initially appears as purple papules which enlarge and break down to become deep, necrotic ulcers with a dark red border. Pyoderma gangrenosum is most common on the legs, but can develop anywhere.

Vitiligo, from Latin *vitium* = mark, blemish.

5. ABDOMINAL PAIN (7)

E – Subphrenic abscess

Intra-abdominal abscesses may follow perforation of a viscus (peptic ulcer, appendix), surgery, and penetrating abdominal injuries. Localized collections of pus may occur around inflamed or infected organs, or free fluid may track and collect in potential spaces within the abdomen (below the diaphragm, within the pelvis, paracolic gutters, lesser sac). Symptoms may be insidious and include pain, tenderness, swinging fevers, and generalized weakness.

A subphrenic abscess is a localized collection of pus beneath the diaphragm. It most commonly occurs on the right side. It develops 2–3 weeks following a peritonitic event and apart from the symptoms described above, there may be complaints of shoulder tip pain, hiccups (secondary to diaphragmatic irritation), and respiratory difficulty caused by pulmonary collapse and effusions. A chest X-ray will show fluid under the diaphragm and diagnosis may be confirmed by ultrasound or CT. Treatment is with systemic antibiotics and drainage (either percutaneous or open). Specific features of a pelvic abscess include diarrhoea with tenesmus, urinary frequency and mucous rectal discharge. Subphrenic and pelvic abscesses are usually caused by the tracking of fluid into these potential spaces in a supine patient. Appendix and diverticular abscesses develop following localized perforations. They present with localized symptoms. Rarely, fluid from an infected diverticulum may track into the groin mimicking a strangulated inguinal hernia. *Polycystic liver disease* is an autosomal dominant condition that is associated with polycystic kidneys. The majority of patients are asymptomatic and cysts are found incidentally on ultrasound. Symptoms that do occur are the result of pressure effects from an enlarged multicystic liver and include abdominal pain, back pain, and abdominal distension.

6. GLASGOW COMA SCORE (1)

C – 8

Based on the score (described below), this girl's score is E2 V2 M4, a total of 8.

The Glasgow coma scale (GCS) is a widely used subjective scale for the initial and continuing assessment of conscious levels in patients presenting to the accident and emergency department, particularly in the case of head injury and trauma. It is made up of three components:

Best eye response (E)
- 4   Eyes open spontaneously
- 3   Eyes open to speech
- 2   Eyes open to pain
- 1   No eye opening

Best verbal response (V)
- 5   Coherent speech
- 4   Confused/disorientated speech
- 3   Inappropriate words without conversational exchange
- 2   Incomprehensible sounds
- 1   No verbal response

Best motor response (M)
- 6   Obeys commands
- 5   Localizes to pain

4   Withdraws from pain
3   Abnormal flexion in response to pain (decorticate response)
2   Abnormal extension in response to pain (decerebrate response)
1   No motor response

The maximum score is 15 (E4, V5, M6) and the minimum is 3 (E1, V1, M1). Head injuries can be classified on the basis of the GCS as:

Mild   GCS ≥ 13
Moderate   GCS 9–12
Severe   GCS ≤ 8

A GCS of 8 or below is termed coma, and urgent anaesthetic input is required for airway assessment and consideration of intubation.

The scale was first published in 1974 by Teasdale and Jennett, two professors of neurosurgery at the University of Glasgow.

7. ABDOMINAL PAIN (8)

C – Meckel diverticulitis

A Meckel diverticulum is a congenital diverticulum, an embryonic remnant of the omphalomesenteric duct, which contains gastric-type mucosa. It is an example of a true diverticulum. A true diverticulum incorporates all the layers of the wall from which it arises. Conversely, a false diverticulum is made up of only the inner layer of the normal bowel wall, an example being colonic diverticula. There is a rule of '2's surrounding the Meckel diverticulum: it is found 2 feet proximal to the ileo-caecal junction, it is 2 inches in length and it occurs in 2% of the population. Most Meckel diverticula are incidental findings, but the most common presentation is painless rectal bleeding. Some may present with an acute inflammation that is clinically similar to acute appendicitis, but may include per rectum bleeding. Because Meckel diverticula contain gastric mucosa, they are susceptible to peptic ulceration. Diagnosis is confirmed by a ^{99}Technetium scan. The radio-labelled technetium is only taken up by gastric-type mucosa, so the scan will highlight the stomach as well as a diverticulum in the right iliac fossa. Treatment is by resection if required.

Diverticulum, from Latin *diverticulum* = by road.

Johann Friedrich Meckel, German anatomist (1781–1833).

8. DYSPHAGIA (3)

D – Pharyngeal pouch

A pharyngeal pouch (or Zenker diverticulum) develops from the backward protrusion of mucosa between the inferior constrictor and cricopharyngeus muscles of the pharynx (known as Killian dehiscence). The pouch formed by the protruding mucosa initially develops posteriorly but may later protrude to one side, usually the left, displacing the oesophagus laterally. Pharyngeal pouches are uncommon before the age of 70 and are five times more common in men. Presentation is with dysphagia, regurgitation of pouch contents, halitosis, recurrent aspiration, night-time coughing and a neck swelling in the anterior triangle which gurgles on palpation. The pouch is easily visualized on barium swallow and management is by surgical excision of the pouch. Note that care must be taken when performing an endoscopy on these patients as there is a risk of perforating the pouch.

A *laryngocoele* is an air-filled sac that communicates with the larynx. It may be present as a congenital abnormality or arise secondary to raised pressures in the laryngeal ventricle, e.g. in chronic obstructive pulmonary disease (COPD) or players of wind instruments. If the laryngocoele is limited to the paraglottic space (internal) it presents with stridor and hoarseness; if it protrudes through the thyrohyoid membrane, it presents as a reducible lump in the anterior triangle of the neck, which recurs on coughing, sneezing, etc.

The anterior triangle is the area that is bounded medially by the midline of the neck, laterally by the anterior border of the sternocleidomastoid and at its base by the lower border of the mandible. All the differentials listed above may present as a lump in the anterior triangle of the neck.

Gustav Killian, German laryngologist (1860–1921).

Friedrich von Zenker, German physician (1825–1898).

9. FLUID THERAPY (2)

C – Gelofusin

The most commonly used fluids in practice are the crystalloids and the colloids. Crystalloids are solutions of water-soluble molecules which are able to pass through a semi-permeable membrane. Examples of crystalloids include normal saline, 5% dextrose and Hartmann solution. Colloids are made up of larger insoluble molecules and hence stay in the circulation for longer; examples include Gelofusin and Haemaccel. Blood is a naturally occurring colloid. In the setting of acute trauma, the fluids given depend largely on what is to hand, but if there is a clinical suspicion of haemorrhage and packed red cells are available, then they should be given, preferably typed and cross-matched, unless it is acutely-life threatening in which case O negative blood may be used. Fresh frozen plasma contains only the plasma portion of blood and is used to correct abnormal coagulation, including rapidly reversing the effects of warfarin and treating deficiencies of clotting factors. Mannitol is a plant-derived sugar alcohol. It is used clinically as an osmotic diuretic in certain cases of raised intracranial pressure, although its role is controversial.

10. MANAGING ANORECTAL DISEASE (3)

E – Seton insertion

This man has probably developed an anal fistula as a complication of inflammatory bowel disease. A fistula is defined as an abnormal connection between two epithelial surfaces. The only exception to this is an arteriovenous fistula which is a connection between two endothelial surfaces. An anal fistula results when an anal abscess ruptures into the anal canal. Patients present with a constant discharge from the external opening of the fistula. Goodsall's rule can be applied to the examination of anal fistulae. It states that if a fistula lies in the anterior half of the anal area then it opens directly into the anal canal. However, if it lies in the posterior half, then the fistula tracks around the anus to open in the midline posteriorly. The best way to delineate the anatomy of a fistula is by MRI scanning.

The treatment of anal fistula depends on whether or not it passes through the puborectalis muscle of the anal sphincter. Inter-sphincteric fistulae (that lie below puborectalis) are managed by laying open the fistula tract. Higher trans-sphincteric fistulae (which pass through puborectalis) should not be laid open due to the significant risk of subsequent faecal incontinence. Instead a non-absorbable suture (or seton) is passed into the fistula tract and tied. This gradually cuts through the muscle allowing it to heal by scarring.

11. ANATOMY OF HERNIAS (1)

C – Lumbar hernia

There are two types of lumbar hernia. A Petit hernia (as in this question) passes through the inferior lumbar triangle of the posterolateral wall, which is bounded by external oblique, latissimus dorsi and the iliac crest below. A Grynfeltt hernia passes through the superior lumbar triangle, a space bounded by the 12th rib above, sacrospinalis muscle medially and the internal oblique muscle laterally.

For a description of the other listed hernias, see the question, 'Anatomy of hernias (3)'.

Jean Louis Petit, French surgeon (1674–1750).

Joseph Grynfeltt, French surgeon (1840–1913).

12. TESTICULAR DISEASE

E – Testicular cancer

Testicular cancer is the most common cancer affecting men between the ages of 20 and 40. It accounts for up to 2% of malignancies in men. Most testicular tumours are germ cell tumours (95%) – seminomas and teratomas. Tumours in older men (>60 years) tend to be lymphomas. The biggest risk factor for the development of testicular cancer is an undescended testis, with the risk increased 30-fold. The risk remains unchanged even after orchidopexy; this procedure just enables any abnormality to be detected early. Presentation of tumours is usually with a painless, irregular lump in the testis or as testicular enlargement. Other symptoms include haematospermia, pain in the scrotum and a secondary hydrocele. On examination, it is possible to 'get above' the lump. Diagnosis of a tumour is made on ultrasound but the type of tumour is only established following orchidectomy and histological evaluation (biopsies are not performed due to the risk of seeding). CT is used to look for metastasis. Treatment involves orchidectomy, with adjuvant radiotherapy for seminomas, orchemotherapy for non-seminomas. The overall prognosis of localized disease is good (95% at 5 years). Teratomas have a poorer prognosis as they metastasize early (by haematogenous spread).

A *haematocele* is a collection of blood within the tunica vaginalis. It usually follows trauma and presents with pain, but may also occur spontaneously from underlying disease of the testis. Initially the swelling is fluctuant but later becomes firm. *Epididymal cyst* presents as a painless swelling on the upper pole of the testis. On palpation, the mass is separate from the testis, is fluctuant and transilluminates. Cysts are more common after middle age and may be bilateral. *Orchitis* (inflammation of the testis) presents with a painful swollen testicle. The majority of cases are viral in origin. A *gumma* is a granuloma. They may occur on the testis in tertiary syphilis.

13. BREAST DISEASE (3)

D – Paget disease

Paget disease of the nipple is an eczema-like (i.e. dry and itchy) condition of the nipple which persists despite local treatment and is associated with an underlying breast carcinoma. As the disease progresses, the nipple erodes and eventually disappears. The diagnosis of Paget disease is confirmed by biopsy of the lesion.

Mondor disease is a rare condition describing thrombophlebitis of the superficial veins of the breast and anterior chest wall. It is characterized by a painful, inflamed subcutaneous cord which is tethered to the skin. When the arm on the affected side is raised, a shallow groove becomes apparent alongside the cord. Treatment is with rest and analgesia.

Henri Mondor, French surgeon (1885–1962).

Sir James Paget, English surgeon (1814–1899).

14. INVESTIGATING DYSPHAGIA (3)

C – Neck, chest and abdominal X-rays

It is not uncommon for young children to be brought to hospital after having swallowed a foreign body. The most common age group involved are children under the age of 5. Commonly swallowed objects include coins, pins, small toys and batteries. The majority of swallowed objects will pass uneventfully through the gastrointestinal tract and exit via the faeces, however all patients presenting with such a history must be investigated, due to potential complications. Complications caused by foreign objects include airway obstruction, gastrointestinal obstruction, perforation and erosion, so the child must be carefully assessed for any signs of these. In the majority of cases, objects which have passed through the lower oesophageal sphincter and into the stomach will make it through the rest of the tract. In the first instance, in a stable child who has swallowed a radio-opaque object, perform a neck, chest and abdominal film to confirm the presence and location of a foreign body. If the position of the object is below the gastric cardia, the child can then be monitored with serial X-rays. If the object is not radio-opaque then a CT scan, barium swallow or upper GI endoscopy should be performed. Barium swallows must not be performed however if there is any risk or suspicion of perforation. Indications for an immediate endoscopy include evidence of airway obstruction or other complications, ingestion of potentially harmful objects (batteries, toothpicks) and ingestion of large objects (>6 cm) that are unlikely to pass through the stomach. Direct laryngoscopy may be used to remove foreign bodies lodged in the throat, e.g. fish bones.

15. ENDOCRINE DISEASE (3)

C – Conn syndrome

This man presents with polyuria and polydipsia associated with high sodium, low potassium and normal glucose. This suggests a diagnosis of Conn syndrome.

Conn syndrome results from an aldosterone-secreting adenoma of the adrenal gland. Aldosterone causes sodium reabsorption and potassium excretion in the kidneys. Excess aldosterone results in sodium and water retention leading to a high blood pressure and oedema. Surplus potassium excretion results in hypokalaemia, the features of which include muscle cramps and weakness, polyuria (secondary to renal tubular damage, i.e. nephrogenic diabetes insipidus) and polydipsia. The diagnosis of Conn syndrome can be made by measuring serum aldosterone and renin levels – aldosterone will be raised and renin levels will be reduced due to negative feedback. You should note that many antihypertensive medications interfere with these hormones so it is important to stop these for at least 6 weeks before testing. Initial management is with spironolactone, an aldosterone antagonist. Once the adenoma is localized (using CT) it can be surgically removed.

Jerome Conn, American endocrinologist (1907–1981).

16. INVESTIGATING GI BLEEDING

E – Oesophagogastroduodenoscopy (OGD)

This patient has presented with melaena – black, tarry stools caused by bleeding in the upper intestinal tract (from mouth to duodenum – generally above the ligament of Treitz, a suspensory muscle that connects the distal duodenum to the diaphragm). The black appearance is due to the digestion and oxidization of iron in haemoglobin as it passes through the ileum and colon. This patient is suffering from arthritis and may be taking non-steroidal anti-inflammatories, whose long-term use is associated with peptic ulceration. The site of bleeding from the upper GI tract is best seen on OGD. Although barium studies enable the identification of the structure and motility of the upper GI tract, OGD allows direct visualization and enables intervention at the same time, e.g. injecting a bleeding ulcer. All patients that present with any form of gastrointestinal bleeding must have a full blood count and coagulation screen. Results of the full blood count will give an indication of the severity of the bleed, indicate need for transfusion (note that this patient is symptomatic) and provide a baseline result if there were to be further bleeding. A coagulation screen may reveal a coagulopathy to be the cause of the bleed and help identify whether a patient with an acute haemorrhage has developed disseminated intravascular coagulation (DIC). Faecal occult blood tests are used to detect small amounts of blood in the stool that are not visible to the naked eye. They are currently being used as part of the bowel cancer screening programme.

Melaena, from Latin *melas* = black.

Vaclav Treitz, Czech pathologist (1819–1872).

17. SKIN LESIONS (3)

B – Granuloma annulare

Granuloma annulare is a condition characterized by small reddish papules that are arranged in a ring. It usually occurs on the backs of the hands or feet and is often associated with diabetes mellitus. Granuloma annulare is usually asymptomatic and lesions fade after a year. Although aetiology is unknown it is thought to be due to a T-cell mediated reaction.

Seborrhoeic keratoses (or basal cell papillomas) are common pigmented benign tumours of basal keratinocytes that often occur in large numbers on the face and trunk of elderly people. They are dark, rough and greasy and have a 'stuck on' appearance with a well-defined edge. These lesions have no malignant potential but may be removed by excision, cautery or cryotherapy if the patient wishes.

Lipomas are soft, mobile lesions composed of fatty tissue that are usually painless. The presence of multiple painful lipomas is known as *Dercum disease* (or adiposis dolorosa). This occurs most commonly in obese middle-aged women and may be accompanied by headaches, amenorrhoea and reduced sweating. Simple lipomas can be removed by excision for cosmetic reasons.

Annulare, from Latin *anus* = ring.

Francis Xavier Dercum, American neurologist (1856–1931).

18. INVESTIGATING ENDOCRINE DISEASE (3)

A – 17-hydroxyprogesterone levels

The presentation of clitoromegaly, precocious puberty and accelerated growth in this young girl is indicative of congenital adrenal hyperplasia. Congenital adrenal hyperplasia (CAH) is an autosomal recessive deficiency of the enzyme 21-hydroxylase. This enzyme is required to synthesize mineralocorticoids and glucocorticoids (but not adrenal androgens) from the hormone precursor 17-hydroxyprogesterone. Because there is a lack of mineralocorticoids and glucocorticoids there is no negative feedback on the anterior pituitary, resulting in increased ACTH secretion. The high ACTH then causes an increased secretion of adrenal androgens, since this does not require the deficient hormone. The androgens result in the physical features of CAH, namely ambiguous genitalia, precocious puberty, accelerated growth in childhood and virilization. The diagnosis of CAH is suggested by finding a raised concentration of the precursor 17-hydroxyprogesterone. Treatment is with hydrocortisone and fludrocortisone to replace the deficient steroids.

19. MANAGING SKIN CONDITIONS (1)

C – Oral antibiotics

Impetigo is a superficial skin infection caused by *Staphylococcus* or *Streptococcus*. It generally occurs in children and presents with thin-walled blisters which itch and bleed and have a superficial golden-yellow crust. These lesions eventually heal without scarring. Impetigo is contagious and requires treatment. If there are only a few lesions, treatment is with bactericidal ointment, such as fusidic acid. If there are many lesions, topical therapy would be inappropriate so oral flucloxacillin is given instead.

Impetigo, from Latin *impetere* = to assail; referring to its aggressively contagious nature.

20. NECK LUMPS (3)

C – Chemodectoma

A chemodectoma is a tumour of carotid body chemoreceptors arising in the carotid bifurcation. It is usually benign. Chemodectoma presents as a slowly enlarging neck mass which demonstrates a transmitted carotid pulsation. It characteristically mobilizes side to side but not up and down as the tumour gets caught in the surrounding structures. Pressure on the tumour may cause dizziness and syncope by stimulating vagal tone via the carotid sinus. Diagnosis is by carotid angiogram which shows a highly vascularized tumour at the carotid bifurcation. Treatment of chemodectomas is by surgical excision.

Syncope, from Greek *syncopa* = to cut short.

21. EPISTAXIS

C – Osler-Weber-Rendu syndrome

Nosebleeds (epistaxis) are a common occurrence in the population with a peak incidence in children and then again after the sixth decade. Most bleeds arise from the anterior nasal septum (Kiesselbach's plexus/Little's area). Posterior bleeds arise from the sphenopalatine artery. Causes of epistaxis may be local (trauma, cold, foreign body) or systemic (hypertension, vascular abnormalities and coagulopathies). The appearance of multiple telangiectasias in this patient, together with a family history of epistaxis, suggests a diagnosis of Osler-WeberRendu syndrome.

Osler-Weber-Rendu syndrome is an autosomal dominant condition characterized by telangiectasia and arteriovenous (AV) malformations at multiple sites. It may present at any age, commonly with recurrent epistaxis, which occurs in up to 90% of those affected. Other problems include gastrointestinal bleeding, haemoptysis, respiratory compromise secondary to pulmonary AV malformations and haemorrhagic strokes. Patients may also have neurological features such as headaches and seizures (10%). Treatment is symptomatic and follows the usual course of pressure on the nose, followed by cautery and packing.

Sturge-Weber syndrome is a sporadic congenital neurocutaneous condition characterized by a port wine stain in the distribution of the trigeminal nerve together with neurological abnormalities (learning disabilities, seizures). *Haemophilia B* is an X-linked autosomal recessive condition in which a deficiency of factor IX results in recurrent spontaneous bleeds into soft tissues and joints. Nasal polyps occur in around 5% of the population and are more common in males. They are associated with allergies and infections. *Septal polyps* may bleed and other presenting symptoms include difficulty breathing and postnasal drip. Malignancy must be considered with unilateral polyps. Treatment may be with topical steroids or surgical (polypectomy). Epistaxis is a recognized but rare presentation of hypertension.

Epistaxis, from Greek *epi* = from + *stactic* = drip; 'dripping from', especially with regards to blood from the nose.

22. KNEE CONDITIONS (1)

E – Septic arthritis

Septic arthritis is an orthopaedic emergency caused by suppurative inflammation within the joint space which can rapidly destroy the joint.

It generally affects the knee and hip but can occur in any joint. It can result from haematogenous spread of infection, direct spread (as in a penetrating wound) or from neighbouring infection. The most common infective agent is *Staphylococcus aureus*. If a septic joint is suspected the patient must be admitted immediately and commenced on intravenous antibiotics following joint aspiration. The joint must be formally washed out, either arthroscopically or as an open procedure. All the other differentials in this question can also present as an acutely swollen joint. *Gout* more commonly affects the big toe and is diagnosed by finding negatively birefringent, needle-shaped crystals (sodium urate). *Pseudogout* is caused by deposition of calcium pyrophosphate dihydrate crystals in the joint space. These are positively birefringent on microscopy. *Reiter's syndrome* is the triad of seronegative arthritis, conjunctivitis and urethritis.

23. CHEST TRAUMA (3)

A – Cardiac tamponade

Cardiac tamponade is the clinical syndrome caused by the accumulation of fluid in the pericardial space – in this case blood. The increased pressure within the pericardium reduces ventricular filling and impairs venous return thereby reducing cardiac output. It is a life threatening emergency which can rapidly result in electromechanical dissociation and cardiac arrest. The classic presentation of cardiac tamponade is Beck's triad – hypotension, raised jugular venous pressure (JVP) and muffled heart sounds. Other signs include pulsus paradoxus, increased respiratory rate, Kussmaul's sign (rising of the JVP on inspiration) and decreased consciousness. ECG demonstrates low voltage QRS complexes and ST segment changes. In an acute trauma setting, a pericardiocentesis is performed if cardiac tamponade is suspected. If the procedure is unsuccessful or the patient is rapidly deteriorating, a thoracotomy in the resuscitation room may be required.

　Claude Schaeffer Beck, American surgeon (1894–1971).
　Adolph Kussmaul, German physician (1822–1902).

24. HERNIAS (3)

D – Incisional hernia

Incisional hernias occur through a defect in a scar from a previous operation. Predisposing factors include poor nutrition, obesity, steroids, a chronic cough, poor wound suture technique and infection of the original wound. The neck of such hernias is usually wide so strangulation is rare. Treatment is by dissection and re-suturing of the layers of the abdominal wall, with or without mesh insertion.

　A *hiatus hernia* describes the protrusion of the upper part of the stomach into the thorax through a defect in the diaphragm. There are three types: (1) a sliding hernia (95% of cases) –where the gastro-oesophageal junction (GOJ) gets pulled up into the thorax; (2) a rolling hernia (5%) – where the GOJ remains in place but a portion of the fundus of the stomach herniates adjacent to the GOJ; and (3) a mixed type with elements of both sliding and rolling hernias (rare).

Hiatus hernias are commoner in obese, older women and the majority are asymptomatic. Features of hiatus hernias include acid reflux, waterbrash (reflex salivation secondary to acid reflux into the lower oesophagus), a night cough (due to refluxed acid tracking to the proximal oesophagus on lying down) and dysphagia. A chest X-ray may demonstrate an air–fluid level within the hernia behind the heart, but agastroscopy would be the best determining investigation. Sliding hernias are managed with symptomatic treatments (e.g. proton pump inhibitors). Rolling hiatus hernias require urgent surgical repair due to the risk of a complete gastric volvulus.

Epigastric hernias often occur in middle-aged men following lifting. Herniation occurs through a defect in the linea alba, which runs between the umbilicus and xiphisternum, and begins as a small protrusion of extra-peritoneal fat which gradually enlarges.

25. CERVICAL SPINE MANAGEMENT

C – He has no cervical spine tenderness

The cervical spine may only be 'cleared' clinically if all the following apply: the patient is fully alert and orientated, not under the influence of drugs or alcohol, there is no head injury, no neck pain, no abnormal neurology and no distracting injuries together with no C-spine tenderness, deformity or external evidence of injury on clinical examination. If any of these are present, imaging must be obtained. Remember that life-threatening treatment takes precedence over clearing the spine and can be carried out while the patient is immobilized.

26. PAEDIATRIC ORTHOPAEDICS (3)

A – Developmental dysplasia of the hip

Developmental dysplasia of the hip (DDH; previously known as congenital dislocation of the hip) encompasses a range of disorders ranging from a mildly dysplastic hip to an overtly dislocated one. The primary abnormality is thought to be a shallow and anteverted acetabulum, with anteversion of the femoral head and neck. The overall prevalence of DDH is 3/1000 (higher at birth). It most commonly affects the left hip of girls. Risk factors include being the first born, breech presentation, oligohydramnios and neuromuscular disorders, e.g. cerebral palsy, spina bifida. It is common in cultures where children are swaddled around their mothers.

Neonatal screening for DDH is by two methods: Barlow test (the hip can easily be displaced posteriorly out of the acetabulum on adduction of the leg with posterior pressure) and Ortolani manoeuvre (the femoral head can be reduced back into the acetabulum on abduction of the leg with anterior pressure). These tests are repeated at regular intervals at baby checks up to the age of 1 year. If there is any suspicion of developmental dysplasia, an ultrasound scan (if the child is 4 months or under) or pelvic X-ray is performed to establish the diagnosis. If the diagnosis is not picked up, the child will present later in life with a painless limp, asymmetric skin creases, limited abduction and external rotation, and shortening of the limb. Occasionally DDH may affect both hip joints. In this case the child will have a wide waddling gait with increased lumbar lordosis. If left untreated, DDH will result in osteoarthritic degeneration of the spine in early adulthood. The treatment depends largely upon the age of presentation. At birth DDH can be treated with an abduction splint, up to 6 months with a Pavlik harness (to allow spontaneous reduction of the femoral head) and after that with surgical reduction (open or closed). Reduction of the femoral head is associated with a risk of avascular necrosis.

Genu varum (or bow-legs) is caused by medial angulation of the tibia in relation to the femur. It may be a normal appearance up to the age of 3, but persistence of the appearance should alert to the possibility of a pathological cause e.g. rickets, scurvy and Paget disease. Genu varum may also be seen in jockeys. The reduced joint space between the tibia and femur present in genu varum leads to the development of osteoarthritis in early adulthood. *Genu valgum* (knock knees) is the name given to the appearance of inwardly angled knees when the legs are held straight. Again it is normal in young children but persistence or worsening deformity is associated with rickets and scurvy. In adults it is associated with osteoarthritis and rheumatoid arthritis.

The original Latin words *varus* and *valgus* had the opposite meaning to their modern use in medicine. *Varus* meant 'knock-kneed' and *valgus* meant 'bowlegged', because the Latin words actually described the position of the leg at the hip joint rather than at the knee joint.

Genu, from Latin *genu* = knee.

Marino Ortolani, Italian paediatrician (1904–1983).

Sir Thomas Barlow, English physician and paediatrician (1845–1945).

27. JAUNDICE (3)

C – Gilbert syndrome

This patient's blood results confirm that he has a pre-hepatic jaundice as identified by an isolated raised bilirubin level. Gilbert syndrome is caused by the abnormal uptake of albumin-bound bilirubin by hepatocytes and causes an unconjugated hyperbilirubinaemia. Symptoms are mild and consist of general malaise and mild jaundice, precipitated by fever, stress, exercise and alcohol. Gilbert syndrome is a benign condition and requires no specific treatment.

Type I Crigler–Najjar syndrome is an autosomal recessive cause of pre-hepatic jaundice, characterized by a complete deficiency of the hepatic enzyme glucuronyl transferase. It presents with neonatal jaundice and may result in kernicterus. Treatment is with phototherapy. It has a high mortality rate. In *type II Crigler–Najjar* syndrome there is a partial deficiency of glucuronyl transferase. Jaundice is less marked and patients tend to live to adulthood. In both viral and alcoholic hepatitis there will be an increase in the hepatic enzymes ALT and AST. Gallstones in the common bile duct cause an obstructive jaundice and an elevated alkaline phosphatase will also be present.

Nicolas Augustin Gilbert, French physician (1858–1927).

28. MANAGING UROLOGICAL DISEASE (1)

B – Catheterization using a three-way catheter

This patient has developed urinary retention, most likely secondary to clot retention. He will require catheterization for relief of his symptoms. Although this could be done using a standard Foley catheter, it is best to use a three-way catheter as irrigation of the bladder with normal saline can be performed simultaneously to allow the clearance of clots and prevent blockage of the catheter. Three-way catheters are often inserted routinely in the presence of frank haematuria to prevent clot retention; they may also be used prophylactically when bleeding is expected, e.g. following a transurethral resection of the prostate. Complications of catheter insertion include urethral irritation, urinary tract infections and urethral stricture formation. A complication of continuous bladder irrigation is hyponatraemia (caused by absorption of irrigation fluid). Suprapubic catheterization is only used when urethral catheterization has failed repeatedly or is contraindicated, e.g. following urethral injuries. Suprapubic catheterization is contraindicated in the presence of pelvic or bladder tumours (which may be the cause of haematuria in this scenario), coagulopathies, previous abdominal or pelvic surgery (as the bowel may have become adherent to the bladder or anterior abdominal wall, so risks perforation) and a non-distended bladder. If repeated attempts at urethral catheterization fail and suprapubic catheterization is contraindicated, a catheter may be inserted at cystoscopy or by using an introducer (this should only be performed by experienced hands).

29. GROIN LUMPS (3)

E – Yolk sac carcinoma

The majority of testicular tumours arise from the germ cells (>90%) and are classified as either seminomas (from the sperm-producing cells) or non-seminomas. Non-seminomas are the most common testicular tumour of children, but also have a peak incidence between the ages of 15 and 40 years. Both yolk sac carcinomas and choriocarcinomas are non-seminomas. Yolk sac carcinomas produce alpha fetoprotein and choriocarcinomas produce human chorionic gonadotrophin. These markers are useful in both diagnosis and monitoring the patient post-treatment. Leydig cell tumours are stromal in origin and can produce either excessive testosterone or less commonly oestrogens (leading to feminization). Lymphomas of the testis are secondary tumours and are the most common type of testicular tumour in men over the age of 40.

30. MANAGING BILIARY TRACT DISEASE

B – ERCP

Choledocholithiasis describes a stone in the common bile duct. Patients may be asymptomatic; however, complications may arise, including obstructive jaundice, ascending cholangitis and pancreatitis. A stone that remains in the common bile duct will eventually cause secondary biliary cirrhosis and liver failure. In view of the patient's symptoms, the stone must be removed. The best way to do this is via endoscopic retrograde cholangiopancreatography (ERCP). ERCP involves cannulation of the biliary tree using a duodenoscope. The biliary tree is entered at its distal point via the sphincter of Oddi and a contrast dye injected. A subsequent X-ray image of the biliary tree will detect an abnormality in this area. Apart from being a diagnostic procedure and confirming the presence of the stone, ERCP also enables removal of the stone at the same time. Other therapeutic interventions allowed by ERCP include palliative stent insertion for obstructive malignant disease and dilatation of benign strictures. Complications of ERCP include pancreatitis (2%), septicaemia, bile duct perforation and contrast reactions. If there is no intended therapeutic need for an ERCP and only imaging is required, then magnetic resonance cholangiopancreatography (MRCP) is the initial investigation of choice as it is non-invasive. Stones that are larger than 1.5 cm may require fragmentation to enable removal. Cholecystectomy is performed in cases of symptomatic gallstones and may be performed as an open or laparoscopic procedure. Indications include recurrent attacks of biliary colic and complications such as ascending cholangitis and pancreatitis.

31. INVESTIGATING ABDOMINAL PAIN (3)

E – Mesenteric angiography

This patient has presented with symptoms typical of mesenteric angina: severe, griping abdominal pain 15–45 minutes after eating. The pain reflects mesenteric ischaemia and occurs as a result of vascular stenosis in the mesenteric arteries (commonly the superior mesenteric artery).

It is comparable to angina and intermittent claudication. The risk factors for the development of mesenteric angina are the same as those for atherosclerosis in general. It typically occurs in those over the age of 60 and is three times more common in females. The treatment is largely surgical, options being endarterectomy, bypass and stenting. Medical management includes anticoagulation with warfarin. Acute or acute-on-chronic mesenteric occlusion presents with ischaemic bowel.

Mesentery, from Greek *mesas* = middle + *enteron* = intestine.

32. PENILE CONDITIONS (1)

E – *Treponema pallidum*

This is a classic presentation of primary syphilis. Syphilis is caused by the bacterium *Treponema pallidum* and is spread by sexual contact (it can also be acquired congenitally). There are many stages of syphilis infection. *Primary syphilis* occurs 10–90 days post-infection. A dull, red papule develops on the external genitalia and forms a single, well-demarcated, painless ulcer associated with bilateral inguinal lymph node enlargement. This lesion heals within 8 weeks. *Secondary syphilis* develops 7–10 weeks after primary infection and involves malaise, mild fever, headache, a pruritic skin rash, hoarseness, swollen lymph nodes, patchy or diffuse hair loss, bone pain and arthralgia. *Latent syphilis:* there is no clinical evidence of disease but it is still detectable by serological testing. *Tertiary syphilis* comprises cardiovascular, gummatous and neurological syphilis. *Cardiovascular syphilis* is characterized by aortitis and aortic aneurysms. *Gummatous syphilis* is a late stage of infection when the host resistance to the infection begins to fail. Areas of syphilitic granulation tissue develop on the scalp, upper aspect of the leg or sternoclavicular region. These so-called 'gummatous' lesions are copper in colour. Granulation can also occur internally, e.g. on heart valves and bone. At this stage, there is still a good response to treatment.

Initial diagnosis of syphilis is by dark ground microscopy (which shows the bluish coiled *Treponema* organisms against the dark brown background) and the Venereal Disease Research Laboratory (VDRL) test, which detects the presence of anticardiolipin, an antibody produced by people with syphilis. False positives to the VDRL test can occur with infectious mononucleosis, antiphospholipid syndrome and leprosy. Treatment of syphilis is with benzylpenicillin (or doxycycline if there is a penicillin allergy).

Haemophilus ducreyi is a sexually transmitted bacterium, common in the tropics, that causes chancroid – a condition typified by a painful ulcer and painful lymphadenopathy. Human papilloma virus is the cause of genital warts. Herpes simplex infection of the genitalia presents with multiple painful blisters. *E. coli* is a common cause of urinary tract infection but not of genital lesions.

33. BONE PAIN (1)

C – Prostatic carcinoma

This patient's history of difficulty passing urine together with the presence of an osteosclerotic lesion in the femur is highly suggestive of a diagnosis of metastatic prostate carcinoma. Prostate cancer is the second most common cancer in men and the second leading cause of cancer death in men. The incidence of prostatic carcinoma increases with age (rare before the age of 60) and there is a greater risk in men of Afro-Caribbean origin. Most tumours are adenocarcinomas (95%) and arise in the peripheries of the prostate. The cancer is usually slow-growing and most men remain asymptomatic and die from other causes. More than 50% of those who do present do so with features of metastatic disease. Symptoms of local disease include those of bladder outflow obstruction (most common), haematuria, haematospermia, back pain and constipation. The most common presentation of metastasis is with bone pain or a pathological fracture. The most common sites of bony metastasis are the lumbar spine, proximal femur and pelvis. Bony metastases have an osteosclerotic appearance on X-ray. Examination reveals a hard irregular 'craggy' prostate with loss of the medial sulcus. Diagnosis is made by the presence of an elevated prostate specific antigen (PSA) and with prostate biopsy. Bone scans and CTs are used to establish the spread of the disease. Management is dependent on the extent of disease. Confined disease may be managed on a watch and wait basis (if life expectancy is not more than 10 years and the tumour is not aggressive). Interventional treatment includes radical prostatectomy, brachytherapy (inserting radio-active seeds into the prostate by transrectal ultrasound) and external beam radiotherapy. Treatment of advanced disease includes the use of luteinizing hormone releasing hormone agonists, anti-androgens, bilateral orchidectomy and bisphosphonates. The prognosis of prostate cancer depends on the extent of spread (stage) and the grade of cancer (determined histologically) as recorded by the Gleason score. The higher the Gleason score, the worse the prognosis.

Osteosclerotic lesions are also found with Paget disease and metastatic breast cancer. Prostatitis is an inflammation of the prostate, generally caused by bacterial infection. It may present as an acute condition (requiring urgent treatment) or may take a chronic course. Causes include urinary tract and sexually transmitted infections. Acute prostatitis is a recognized complication of transrectal biopsy of the prostate. Presentation is with fever, dysuria and perineal pain. Treatment is with appropriate antibiotics for at least a month. Chronic non-bacterial prostatitis (also known as chronic pelvic pain syndrome) is a condition of unknown aetiology causing unremitting chronic perineal pain.

34. INVESTIGATING VASCULAR DISEASE (1)

B – 0.3

The ankle brachial pressure index (ABPI) is calculated by taking the greatest of the systolic pressures in either the posterior tibial artery or the dorsalis pedis, and dividing this by the systolic pressure in the brachial artery on the same side. A normal reading should be 1.0 or above. Calcification of arteries, as can occur in diabetes, can give abnormally high readings (>1.3) even in the presence of significant peripheral vascular disease. These patients should be referred for further investigation. Intermittent claudication will give a reading of 0.5 to 1.0, and readings of between 0.3 and 0.5 are expected in those with rest pain. Readings of below 0.2 occur in the acutely ischaemic leg, and those with gangrene and ulcers.

35. ABDOMINAL PAIN (9)

D – Stricture formation

This patient has presented with the signs and symptoms of bowel obstruction, however his background history is suggestive of Crohn disease. Crohn disease is a non-specific inflammatory bowel disease, thought to be of autoimmune pathogenesis. It is characterized histologically by full-thickness inflammation of the bowel and non-caseating granulomas. Mucosal ulceration along with the intermittent oedema that occurs in Crohn disease results in a cobblestone appearance of the bowel. Crohn disease can occur anywhere in the GI tract, from mouth to anus, although 40% of cases affect the terminal ileum. The next most common site is the colon. The disease does not affect the bowel in a continuous manner.

Crohn disease typically presents in young adults (teens to 20s), with an equal incidence in males and females. It is associated with a family history and is more prevalent in smokers. Presenting symptoms include intermittent abdominal pain, diarrhoea and blood in the stools. Those with active disease may also have fevers, anorexia and weight loss. A mass may be palpable in the right iliac fossa, representing the inflamed terminal ileum. Perianal manifestations, such as the development of fissures and skin tags, are relatively common in Crohn disease.

Extra-intestinal manifestations of Crohn disease include mouth ulcers, oxalate renal calculi, arthritis, erythema nodosum and pyoderma gangrenosum. Complications of Crohn include intraluminal stricture formation (caused by recurrent inflammation with scarring) which can cause bowel obstruction. Segments of stricturing can be demonstrated on small bowel enema (string sign of Kantor). Other complications include intra-abdominal abscess formation, fistula formation with the bladder, vagina, etc., malabsorption and an increased risk of bowel cancer.

Primary sclerosing cholangitis is an autoimmune condition in which there is intra-hepatic inflammation of the bile ducts leading to cholestasis and jaundice. *Toxic megacolon* is a life-threatening condition characterized by non-obstructive dilatation of the colon (more than 6 cm on X-ray) together with systemic upset and toxicity. Both of these conditions are associated with inflammatory bowel disease, but are more often seen in those with ulcerative colitis.

Burrill Bernard Crohn, American gastroenterologist (1884–1983).

John Leonard Kantor, American radiologist (1890–1947).

36. HEPATOMEGALY (3)

B – Amoebic liver abscess

The formation of an amoebic liver abscess is a complication caused by *Entamoeba histolytica* infection of the large intestine. *Entamoeba histolytica* is a protozoan infection transmitted by the faeco-oral route. Infection is associated with old age, malnutrition, immunosuppression and travel to the tropics. A history of dysentery may be clear in only around 15% of those who present with an abscess, and an abscess may develop many years after initial infection. The abscess may easily be detected on an abdominal ultrasound or CT. Serology for amoebiasis is positive. Faecal microscopy may reveal trophozoites in active dysentery. The majority of abscesses develop within the right lobe of the liver. Abscesses within the left lobe of the liver may rupture into the pericardium, causing pericarditis (rare). Treatment is with metronidazole and drainage of the abscess.

Pyogenic liver abscesses arise from infection in the portal system or biliary tree (e.g. following appendicitis or a pelvic infection). They may be single or multiple. Clinical features include swinging pyrexia, jaundice and a tender palpable liver. The diagnosis is confirmed by imaging. Treatment is with systemic antibiotics and drainage. Multiple cysts develop within the liver as a feature of adult-onset polycystic disease (another common site is the kidney). Despite the appearance and size of the liver, it functions as normal. Fitz-Hugh–Curtis syndrome is an inflammation of the connective tissue surrounding the liver (Glisson's capsule), secondary to pelvic inflammatory disease. The condition is almost exclusive to women.

37. MANAGEMENT OF ARTERIAL DISEASE (2)

D – Embolectomy

This man has acute limb ischaemia secondary to an embolism, most probably from the atrial fibrillation. An acutely ischaemic limb is a surgical emergency and needs to be resolved within 6 hours to prevent irreversible necrosis. Initial management is with oxygen and intravenous fluids, analgesia and immediate anticoagulation (5000 units of IV heparin). The next stage is to restore arterial continuity.

With embolus-induced ischaemia, management would either be with thrombolysis or surgical embolectomy. Thrombolysis is appropriate if the ischaemia is acute-on-chronic since this means the limb is not too acutely ischaemic and will remain viable for a long enough time to allow clot dissolution thanks to the development of collaterals. In thrombolysis a cannula is inserted into the distal extent of the thrombus and streptokinase or tissue plasminogen activator infused. Clot dissolution may take several hours. Complications of thrombolysis include anaphylaxis and haemorrhage. Contraindications to thrombolysis include recent surgery, recent stroke and bleeding tendencies.

Since this patient has no history of chronic limb ischaemia, a surgical embolectomy would be the management of choice. In this procedure a catheter with a deflated balloon on it (Fogarty catheter) is passed distal to the embolus. The balloon is then inflated and the catheter pulled out, dragging the embolus with it.

38. HAND DISORDERS (1)

C – Mallet finger

Mallet finger (or baseball finger) occurs when sudden passive flexion of a distal interphalangeal (DIP) joint (like a ball striking the tip of the finger) ruptures the extensor tendon at the point of its insertion into the base of the distal phalanx. The DIP joint rests in mid-flexion and cannot be actively extended. The index and ring fingers are most commonly affected. Treatment is by splinting the affected finger with the DIP extended and the PIP flexed, to allow the tendon to reattach.

Trigger finger (digital tenovaginitis stenosans) is caused by thickening and constriction of the mouth of the tendon sheath, which interferes with free movement of the contained flexor tendons, commonly affecting the ring and middle finger. The affected tendon becomes swollen distal to the sheath constriction. This means that it is easy to flex the tendon (as the swollen nodule slides out of the tendon sheath) but difficult to extend the finger without help. The thickening of the sheath forms a palpable nodule at the base of the finger. Treatment is by incising the mouth of the fibrous flexor sheath longitudinally. A boutonniere injury results in *boutonniere deformity,* characterized by flexion at the proximal interphalangeal joint and hyperextension at the distal interphalangeal joint. It is caused by disruption in the attachment of the central slip of the extensor tendon to the base of the middle phalanx, leading to unopposed action of the flexors. It can be caused by forced flexion injuries (with co-existent fractures of the middle phalanx), dislocations and cuts at the PIP joint, and with chronic inflammation such as occurs in rheumatoid arthritis. Treatment is by splinting the PIP joint (while enabling movement at the DIP and MCP joints), or by surgical repair if the injury is open. Note that presentation of such a deformity following injury may be late.

A *swan neck deformity* is characterized by hyperextension at the PIP joint and flexion at the DIP joint. It may be traumatic in origin but is most commonly seen in rheumatoid arthritis. It is caused by stretching of the ligament anterior to the PIP joint (the volar plate); treatment may be surgical or non-surgical (splinting and rehabilitation). The *duck bill deformity* (or Z-deformity) is a similar deformity which affects the thumb; here the IPJ is hyperextended and there is fixed flexion and subluxation at the metacarpophalangeal joint.

39. MANAGING ANORECTAL DISEASE (1)

E – Topical GTN ointment

This patient has presented with an anal fissure. Anal fissures are longitudinal tears in the anal mucosa, with exposure of the underlying circular muscle, and they typically occur on the passage of a constipated stool. Patients present with a stinging pain that can last up to 2 hours on defaecation. This may be associated with a small amount of fresh bleeding and pruritus. Anal fissures most commonly occur posteriorly in the midline – this is an area of relatively poor blood supply in the anus, hence it is more susceptible to ischaemic damage. Anterior tears in women are associated with childbirth, and multiple anal fissures can occur in Crohn disease. Anal fissures in children must alert the clinician to the possibility of sexual abuse. The skin tag that is associated with anal fissures (the sentinel pile) is the torn anal mucosa which is bunched together. Medical treatment with relaxants such as GTN ointment and diltiazem cream aims to relieve pain and aid healing of the fissure. Stool softeners and dietary advice to prevent constipation are also required as anal fissures can be a recurrent problem. Surgical treatment includes sphincterotomy and anal dilatation, although these may result in a degree of incontinence. Chronic recurring fissures may need excision.

40. BACK PAIN (1)

E – Simple analgesia and gentle mobilization

This patient has presented with mechanical back pain which is characteristically worse at the end of the day. He has no other symptoms that would suggest serious pathology, such as neurological symptoms, fever or weight loss. It is reasonable therefore not to carry out any investigation at this stage as very little useful information would be gained (an MRI can be requested if symptoms persist beyond six weeks). Analgesia, such as NSAIDs, can be used in the treatment of mechanical back pain, and gentle mobilization is advised as bed rest often results in stiffness of the back, leading to prolonged symptoms.

41. MANAGING ABDOMINAL PAIN (3)

C – Mesalazine

This patient has presented with ulcerative colitis (UC). Ulcerative colitis is a chronic inflammatory disease of the bowel, characterized by diffuse mucosal inflammation. The condition progresses in a continuous nature from the rectum upwards (unlike Crohn disease where there are intermittent areas of nonaffected bowel). The rectum is always affected and may be the only site of disease (40%), but disease can progress proximally and may affect the entire colon (pan-colitis in 15%). The cause of UC is unknown, although it is thought to be of autoimmune aetiology.

Ulcerative colitis typically presents between the ages of 15 and 40 (with a second peak in the 60s) and has a slight female preponderance. Incidence is greatest in Caucasians and non-smokers. Presenting symptoms include bloody diarrhoea, urgency, tenesmus, weight loss, fevers and malaise. Up to 25% have extraintestinal manifestations of the disease, including osteoporosis, arthritis, primary sclerosing cholangitis, uveitis, erythema nodosum and pyoderma gangrenosum. Diagnosis is made by endoscopy; a biopsy will show inflammation limited to the mucosa and submucosa and the presence of crypt abscesses. UC has a relapsing and remitting course and the treatment depends on disease activity and extent. Proctitis is best treated with aminosalicylates (e.g. mesalazine) which can be administered as a suppository. In more extensive disease these may be given as an enema or orally. Oral steroids (prednisolone) are used in acute attacks of UC (intravenously if there is systemic upset) and in those not controlled by aminosalicylates. Azathioprine (an immune modulator) is used when there is resistance to treatment with steroids. Indications for surgery (colectomy) include uncontrolled disease, active haemorrhage, perforation and toxic megacolon. UC is associated with an increased risk of colon cancer (up to 1% per year) so endoscopic surveillance with biopsy is advised.

42. SPINAL CORD LESIONS (3)

C – Cauda equina syndrome

The spinal cord ends around the level of the junction between L1 and L2. Beyond this lies a bundle-like structure of spinal nerve roots known as the cauda equina. If narrowing of the spinal canal occurs below the level of L2 (for instance in central cord prolapse or from compression by a tumour) then the spinal nerve roots are compromised and the cauda equina syndrome results. Features of cauda equina syndrome include a triad of bowel/bladder disturbance (retention or incontinence), bilateral leg pain and weakness, and loss of sensation in the saddle area (around the perineum). Cauda equina syndrome is considered an emergency and requires urgent decompression either medically or surgically.

Syringomyelia describes the presence of a longitudinal fluid cavity (syrinx) within the spinal cord. These cavities are usually in the cervical segments and disrupt the spinothalamic tracts. Patients present in their 20s to 30s with a segmental dissociated loss of spinothalamic function (i.e. spinothalamic function above and below the lesion is preserved). Dorsal column and motor function remain intact. When a syrinx affects the brainstem, the condition is called syringobulbia. Diagnosis of syringomyelia is by MRI and management is by surgical decompression of the syrinx.

Syringomyelia may be associated with an Arnold-Chiari malformation, congenital herniation of the cerebellar tonsils through the foramen magnum at the base of the skull. Syringomyelia may also be caused by tumours of, or trauma to, the spinal cord.

Syrinx, from Greek *syringx* = tube. The word 'syringe' also derives from this.

Julius Arnold, German pathologist (1835–1915).

Hans Chiari, German pathologist (1851–1916).

43. MANAGING BREAST CANCER

A – Mastectomy

Surgery is the first-line treatment for breast carcinoma. Breast-conserving surgery (i.e. wide local excision) should be used where possible, although a mastectomy is required if the tumour is >4 cm in size. If a patient is keen for breast-conserving therapy but has a tumour that is larger than 4 cm, a course of neo-adjuvant (i.e. pre-surgery) chemotherapy can be tried. This has the effect of reducing the tumour size, and may result in a tumour that is small enough to undergo wide local excision.

Mastectomy is preferable *over* wide local excision if the tumour is >4 cm, is multi-focal or is centrally situated. A modified radical mastectomy involves the removal of the breast, the overlying skin (including the nipple) and the axillary contents. For comparison, a radical mastectomy (unmodified) involves the removal of the pectoralis muscles in addition to the structures listed above.

Ipsilateral radiotherapy is given to all patients who have undergone breast conserving surgery in order to decrease the risk of local recurrence. Radiotherapy may also be given after mastectomy for patients who have a high risk of local recurrence (i.e. large, poorly-differentiated tumours or having more than three positive axillary lymph nodes).

Chemotherapy can be given in some cases of breast cancer. It is considered in premenopausal women who have node-positive disease, or in pre-menopausal women who have node-negative disease but a poorly differentiated (grade III) tumour. A typical chemotherapy regimen is CMF (cyclophosphamide, methotrexate and 5-fluorouracil) given in six cycles every 3 weeks.

Trastuzumab (Herceptin™) is a monoclonal antibody that binds with the Her-2 receptor that may be found within some breast tumours. Activation of the Her-2 receptor results in an arrest in the growth phase of mitosis, so there is reduced proliferation. Trastuzumab is only effective in tumours that express the Her-2 receptor. In pre-menopausal and post-menopausal women with oestrogen receptor-positive tumours, tamoxifen is the hormonal therapy of choice. (Tamoxifen is a selective oestrogen receptor modulator which inhibits the action of oestrogen on the tumour.) In cases where tamoxifen is contraindicated (e.g. a history of venous thromboembolism) an aromatase inhibitor (e.g. anastrozole) is given instead. Arimidex inhibits the peripheral conversion of androgens to oestrogen by aromatase, an enzyme found in body fat. Aromatase inhibitors are only effective in post-menopausal women. This is because pre-menopausal women secrete large amounts of oestrogen from the ovaries and peripheral oestrogen synthesis accounts for only a small amount of total body oestrogen.

44. FOOT DISORDERS (3)

B – Achilles tendon rupture

The Achilles tendon is the largest tendon in the body, connecting the muscles of the calf (gastrocnemius and soleus) to the calcaneum. Rupture most commonly occurs during sporting activities and presents as a sudden pain in the back of the calf or ankle and the sensation of a 'pop' with associated swelling. There will be an inability to stand on tiptoes. Examination will reveal a 'dip' in the region of the rupture and, if the corresponding calf is squeezed, the foot will not plantarflex (Simmonds or Thompson test). Diagnosis may be confirmed on ultrasound or MRI. Treatment may be conservative (plaster cast) or surgical, by suturing the opposed ends of the tendon.

Achilles tendonitis is inflammation of the Achilles tendon caused by repetitive stress, e.g. in athletes. It causes pain on activity. The tendon will be tender and warm, and nodules may be palpable over it. Treatment is with rest and anti-inflammatories. Achilles tendonitis predisposes to rupture. The *posterior cruciate ligament* is one of the four ligaments that stabilizes the knee. Rupture presents with acute knee swelling and instability. The integrity of the ligament is assessed by the posterior draw test. *Calcaneal spurs* are bony projections that develop at the calcaneum. They may be asymptomatic and found incidentally on X-ray. They cause heel pain on walking and may predispose to the development of Achilles tendonitis. Treatment is largely symptomatic. Calcaneal fractures are high-velocity injuries, most commonly caused by axial loading as in a fall from a height onto the feet.

45. THYROID DISEASE (3)

B – Graves disease

This woman demonstrates features of thyrotoxicosis with a thyroid bruit. The presence of hyperthyroidism with a bruit indicates a likely diagnosis of Graves disease. Graves disease is an autoimmune condition resulting in over-activity of the thyroid. The hyperthyroidism is due to the presence of antibodies that stimulate the TSH receptor, resulting in a high secretion of thyroid hormones. Apart from the generic features of thyrotoxicosis (such as diarrhoea, feeling warm, weight loss despite a good appetite, tremor), patients with Graves disease may also demonstrate a thyroid bruit, pretibial myxoedema and ophthalmoplegia. Specific examples of eye disease in Graves disease are lid retraction and proptosis (a 'bulging' appearance of the eyes due to myxoedematous infiltration of the muscles behind the eye). Treatment options for hyperthyroidism include carbimazole, ^{131}iodine and subtotal thyroidectomy. Beta-blockers, such as propranolol, help diminish the symptoms of thyrotoxicosis but do not affect the underlying disease.

Multinodular goitres are most common in middle-aged women. They can present in many ways, including with an unsightly swelling or dysphagia. In some cases, one nodule in a multinodular goitre will become an autonomous thyroxine-secreting adenoma, resulting in features of hyperthyroidism. This scenario is known as a toxic multinodular goitre, or 'Plummer disease'. Cardiac features, such as atrial fibrillation and palpitations, often predominate in toxic multinodular goitre. Treatment is with radio-iodine or subtotal thyroidectomy (anti-thyroid medications such as carbimazole have little effect).

A *thyroid storm* describes a sudden surge in circulating thyroid hormones. It can be precipitated by infection or stress. Patients present with fever, tachycardia, agitation, atrial fibrillation and heart failure. Treatment is in intensive care with fluids, gentle cooling and intravenous beta-blockers (propranolol). Sodium iopodate (which inhibits thyroxine release) and carbimazole (inhibits synthesis of thyroxine) are also administered. Mortality is around 10%.

Robert James Graves, Irish physician (1797–1853).
Henry Stanley Plummer, American physician (1874–1937).

46. SALTER–HARRIS FRACTURES

D – Salter–Harris IV

The Salter–Harris classification describes fractures that involve the growth plate in children. The classification can be remembered using the initials SALTeR:

I	Slipped	Fracture across the physis with no other fragment
II	Above	Fracture across the physis with a metaphyseal fragment

III	Lower	Fracture across the physis with an epiphyseal fragment
IV	Through	Fracture through the physis with metaphyseal + epiphyseal fragments
V	Rammed	Crush injury to the physis

Remember that the metaphysis is the area of bone on the inside of the physis (growth plate) and the epiphysis is the outermost part of the bone.

47. PAEDIATRIC SURGICAL MANAGEMENT (3)

C – Contact the anaesthetist on call and ask them to attend urgently

This child has presented with epiglottitis, an acute bacterial infection of the epiglottis most commonly caused by *Haemophilus influenzae* type B. It most commonly presents between the ages of 2 and 7 but may also affect adults. Initial symptoms include a sore throat, but disease is rapidly progressive and the patient quickly becomes septic, with drooling and difficulty breathing secondary to airway compromise. Epiglottitis is therefore an emergency. Although diagnosis may be made by laryngoscopy, manipulation of the airway may trigger laryngospasm and therefore an anaesthetist must be at hand. Endotracheal intubation may be required if airway compromise is imminent. An enlarged epiglottis may be seen on a lateral soft tissue neck X-ray but this is not a routinely helpful examination. If epiglottitis is suspected, then treatment must be commenced on clinical grounds with intravenous antibiotics.

48. BURNS (1)

D – 27%

Assessing the extent of burns is done quickly using Wallace's 'rule of nines'. The body is divided into units divisible by nine as follows:

Head + neck	→	9%	
Upper limb	→	9% each	
Anterior torso	→	18%	
Posterior torso	→	18%	
Lower limb	→	18% each	
Perineum	→	1%	(Total 100%)

In this example: left arm = 9% and back = 18%, giving a total of 27% burns. All depths of burns are included in assessing extent, regardless of the severity.

An alternate way of assessing the extent of the burn is to take the patient's palm to represent 1% and calculate burn surface area this way.

Although the rule of nines is useful for adults, it is not accurate for children due to the relative disproportionate size of certain body parts. Most burns units have charts (such as the Lund and Browder chart) which can more accurately predict body surface areas with respect to age.

49. LOWER LIMB NERVE LESIONS (3)

E – Tibial nerve

The tibial nerve is particularly vulnerable to damage during posterior dislocations of the knee. It can also be compressed in the posterior tarsal tunnel behind the medial malleolus. A branch of the sciatic nerve, the tibial nerve supplies the flexor compartment of the leg (calf muscles). It also gives rise to the medial and lateral plantar nerves which supply the intrinsic muscles of the foot as well as plantar sensation. Tibial nerve palsy results in loss of toe flexion, ankle inversion and the ankle jerk. Sensation over the plantar surface of the foot is lost. Affected patients walk with a shuffling gait as the take-off phase of walking is impaired. There is loss of the lateral longitudinal arch of the foot, and atrophy of the intrinsic foot muscles eventually results in a claw foot.

Tibia, from Latin *tibia* = shinbone or flute; so-called because it is thought that flutes were once fashioned from the tibia of animals.

50. PAEDIATRIC SURGERY (3)

E – Mesenteric adenitis

Mesenteric adenitis is the term given to the non-specific inflammation of mesenteric lymph nodes, resulting in mild peritoneal irritation. Mesenteric adenitis usually follows a viral infection. Other causative pathogens include *Yersinia enterolytica* and *Campylobacter jejuni*. Mesenteric adenitis is rare after the age of 30 and is most common in children following an upper respiratory tract infection. The presentation of mesenteric adenitis often mimics acute appendicitis; features that may be helpful in differentiating the two are a high grade fever (greater than 38.5°C), shifting tenderness, lack of rebound tenderness and absence of anorexia in mesenteric adenitis. The two conditions are often difficult to differentiate and the diagnosis may sometimes only be made after laparotomy or laparoscopy, on finding a normal appendix and enlarged mesenteric lymph nodes. Mesenteric adenitis is a self-limiting condition and treatment is conservative and symptomatic (analgesia, anti-pyretics).

Coeliac disease is an enteropathy of the small intestine caused by gluten sensitivity. It is the gliadin portion of gluten that stimulates a cell-mediated response, resulting in the destruction of villi and malabsorption. Coeliac disease is most common in the West (with an estimated incidence of 1/100 in the UK) and presentation is usually in the first few years of life with a second peak in middle age. Symptoms include diarrhoea, abdominal distension and a failure to thrive. Diagnosis is made by a combination of blood tests (e.g. for anti-tissue transglutaminase antibodies and anti-gliadin antibodies) and jejunal biopsy. Treatment is with a gluten-free diet. Dermatitis herpetiformis (a blistering, itchy rash affecting the extensor surfaces) is an extra-intestinal manifestation of coeliac disease.

Practice Paper 4: Questions

1. BONE PAIN (2)

A 65-year-old man presents to the GP surgery complaining of increasing pain in his back and lower left leg. His mobility is now very limited. On examination, he has a marked kyphosis of the spine and bowing of the left lower limb. Locally the leg is markedly warm. Blood tests are taken.

Which of the following biochemical abnormalities would one expect to find?

A. Hypercalcaemia and hyperphosphataemia
B. Hypocalcaemia and hypophosphataemia
C. Hypocalcaemia and raised alkaline phosphatase
D. Raised alkaline phosphatase and normal calcium
E. Reduced parathyroid hormone levels and normal calcium

2. MANAGING DYSPHAGIA

A 33-year-old woman presents to the surgical outpatient clinic with increasing dysphagia for solids and liquids, retrosternal chest pain on eating, regurgitation of undigested food and weight loss. Oesophageal and gastric biopsy at endoscopy was normal. Oesophageal manometry showed impaired relaxation of the lower oesophageal sphincter and barium swallow revealed a dilated proximal oesophagus with distal narrowing.

Which of the following surgical procedures would be indicated?

A. Billroth I
B. Billroth II
C. Heller myotomy
D. Ramstedt procedure
E. Whipple procedure

3. BURNS (2)

A 24-year-old man was involved in a house fire and is brought to the emergency department. He has partial thickness burns over the whole of his front torso and right arm, and superficial burns on his left hand.

Estimate the percentage burn he has sustained.

A. 18%
B. 25%
C. 28%
D. 36%
E. 37%

4. FEMORAL NECK FRACTURES (1)

A 45-year-old man is brought to the emergency department having fallen off a ladder. He complains of pain in the right hip. He is normally fit and well. Hip X-rays show a displaced intracapsular fracture.

Which of the following is the best treatment option?

A. Conservative management
B. Dynamic hip screw
C. Hemiarthroplasty
D. Reduction and internal fixation
E. Total hip replacement

5. LOWER LIMB NERVE LESIONS (4)

An 18-year-old boy is attacked in a bar fight, during which he is stabbed in the right groin. He attends the emergency department as he is unable to extend his knee afterwards. On examination, the right knee jerk is absent and there is loss of sensation over the front of the thigh and medial aspect of the leg.

Which nerve has most likely been affected?

A. Common peroneal nerve
B. Femoral nerve
C. Obturator nerve
D. Sciatic nerve
E. Tibial nerve

6. LOCAL ANAESTHETIC AGENTS (1)

A 23-year-old man attends the emergency department after smashing his hand through a window. He has sustained a small laceration to his distal left index finger which you decide to suture.

Which would be the most appropriate anaesthetic agent to use?

A. Bupivacaine
B. Cocaine
C. Lidocaine alone
D. Lidocaine/prilocaine mixture
E. Lidocaine with adrenaline

7. X-RAY APPEARANCES OF GASTROINTESTINAL DISEASE

A 59-year-old woman with a long history of constipation presents with a 4-month history of episodic left-sided abdominal pain relieved by defaecation. She has also had two episodes of fresh bleeding per rectum. There is no history of weight loss and she is otherwise well. Examination is unremarkable. She is referred for a barium enema.

What features would you expect to find?

A. Apple-core lesion
B. Birds beak appearance
C. Diverticular outpouchings
D. Non-filling of the appendix
E. Thumb printing of the colon

8. ABDOMINAL PAIN (10)

A 69-year-old man presents to the GP with a 2-month history of epigastric pain. He also feels full after eating small amounts of food and has lost a stone in weight over the last 2 months. Examination is unremarkable.

Which of the following is the most likely diagnosis?

A. Duodenal ulcer
B. Gastric cancer
C. Gastric ulcer
D. Menetrier disease
E. Pernicious anaemia

9. DYSPHAGIA (4)

A 56-year-old woman presents with progressive difficulty swallowing. She has also noticed increased difficulty in articulating her speech. On examination, you notice that her tongue is small and stiff. She has an exaggerated gag reflex.

Which of the following is the most likely cause of her symptoms?

A. Bulbar palsy
B. Myasthenia gravis
C. Paralysis of the vocal cords
D. Pseudobulbar palsy
E. Scleroderma

10. MANAGING ENDOCRINE DISEASE (1)

A 58-year-old woman is brought to the emergency department having been found unresponsive by her husband at home. On examination, you note that she is overweight with coarse features. Observations include heart rate 42/min, blood pressure 100/68 mmHg and temperature 34.6°C.

Which of the following would be the most appropriate next step in your management?

A. Intravenous thyroxine
B. Intravenous propranolol
C. Oral propylthiouracil
D. Oral thyroxine
E. Thyroidectomy

11. JAUNDICE (4)

A 52-year-old man is brought into hospital by his wife with a 2-day history of confusion. On examination, he is jaundiced and has a distended abdomen with dilated veins around his umbilicus.

Which of the following is the most likely cause of his jaundice?

A. Alcoholic liver disease
B. Autoimmune hepatitis
C. Hepatitis A
D. Hepatitis B
E. Reye syndrome

12. ABNORMAL GLUCOSE METABOLISM

A 42-year-old woman presents with episodes of severe hunger despite regular meals. She states that if she does not eat she becomes sweaty and agitated. Her symptoms are exacerbated by exercise. As a result of needing to eat so regularly she has gained a lot of weight.

Which of the following blood results would correlate with her symptoms?

A. Decreased insulin levels
B. Increased C-peptide levels
C. Increased glucagon levels
D. Increased somatostatin levels
E. Raised fasting blood glucose

13. PENILE CONDITIONS (2)

A 4-year-old boy is brought to the urology clinic by his mother. She is concerned as he is having difficulty urinating properly and is causing a mess. He is otherwise growing and developing normally. On examination, you see the urethral meatus is present on the shaft of the underside of the penis.

Which of the following treatment options would you recommend?

A. Antibiotics
B. Circumcision
C. Intracavernosal injection of phenylephrine
D. Referral to a specialist for corrective surgery
E. Steroid cream

14. PAEDIATRIC SURGERY INVESTIGATION

A 3-day-old boy is having increasing abdominal distension and vomiting. He is also noted not to have passed meconium since birth.

Which of the following investigations would be most helpful in confirming the cause of obstruction?

A. Abdominal X-ray
B. Barium enema
C. Rectal biopsy
D. Rectal examination
E. Ultrasound scan

15. EPONYMOUS FRACTURES (1)

A 13-year-old girl presents to the emergency department following a fall on the outstretched hand. An X-ray of the affected upper limb shows a fracture of the upper ulna with dislocation of the radial head.

Which of the following would be the most appropriate term to describe this fracture?

A. Barton fracture
B. Colles fracture
C. Galeazzi fracture
D. Monteggia fracture
E. Smith fracture

16. ABDOMINAL PAIN (11)

A 35-year-old woman presents to the emergency department with a 1-day history of colicky central abdominal pain and vomiting. She last opened her bowels 2 days ago. She has no past medical history of note but tells you she had an operation on her abdomen as a child although she is not sure what this was for. On examination, she looks unwell and moderately dehydrated. The abdomen is distended and tender with hyperactive bowel sounds.

Which of the following is most likely to have caused her symptoms?

A. Adhesions
B. Colorectal tumour
C. Constipation
D. Gallstone ileus
E. Paralytic ileus

17. ANORECTAL DISEASE (3)

A 36-year-old man complains of a 6-month history of intermittent pain in the rectum which is unrelated to stools. The pain tends to occur at night. He denies passing any mucus or blood per rectum and examination is unremarkable.

Which of the following is the most likely diagnosis?

A. Anal fissure
B. Anal fistula
C. Perianal abscess
D. Perianal haematoma
E. Proctalgia fugax

18. ANATOMY OF HERNIAS (2)

Which term best fits the description of the hernia given below?

A hernia that has two parts, each lying either side of the inferior epigastric artery.

A. Gluteal
B. Lumbar
C. Maydl
D. Obturator
E. Pantaloon

19. AIRWAY MANAGEMENT (1)

A 50-year-old woman has been hit by a car and thrown 5 metres. There was probable loss of consciousness for a few minutes. She is brought in by ambulance, immobilized. On arrival she is alert, orientated and talking happily. Within a few minutes however she starts to deteriorate rapidly and becomes unconscious with a Glasgow coma score of 5.

Which of the following measures is needed to maintain her airway?

A. Endotracheal intubation
B. Hyperextend the neck
C. Nasopharyngeal airway
D. Oropharyngeal airway
E. Supplemental oxygen

20. GROIN LUMPS (4)

A 48-year-old-woman presents with a long-standing, painless swelling on her right thigh which disappears on lying flat. She is otherwise well. On examination, the swelling is bluish and non-pulsatile. It lies below and lateral to the pubic tubercle.

What is the most likely diagnosis?

A. Femoral hernia
B. Inguinal hernia
C. Psoas abscess
D. Saphena varix
E. Sebaceous cyst

21. INVESTIGATING ABDOMINAL PAIN (4)

A 29-year-old woman presents to the emergency department with a 3-hour history of lower abdominal pain. On examination, there is marked rebound tenderness in the left iliac fossa. She has a heart rate of 92/min and a blood pressure of 134/92 mmHg.

Which of the following investigations would you perform in the first instance?

A. Abdominal ultrasound
B. Abdominal X-ray
C. Cervical swabs
D. Urine dipstick
E. Urine pregnancy test

22. KNEE CONDITIONS (2)

A 27-year-old man presents to the emergency department with sudden-onset pain and swelling in his right knee which occurred while walking. He denies any trauma to the knee. The man describes his knee 'locking' at the time, although this sensation is not present now.

What is the most likely diagnosis?

A. Anterior cruciate ligament injury
B. Chondromalacia patellae
C. Osgood–Schlatter disease
D. Osteochondritis dissecans
E. Pre-patellar bursitis

23. INVESTIGATING BREAST DISEASE (1)

A 28-year-old woman comes to see you at the GP practice having noticed a lump in the right breast. She is concerned that it may be cancer. On examination, you find a smooth, mobile, non-tender mass around 2 cm in diameter in the upper outer quadrant of the breast. There are no overlying skin changes.

Which would be the most appropriate action to take?

A. Advise the patient to return if the lump gets bigger or starts becoming painful
B. Prescribe antibiotics
C. Reassure the patient that there is no evidence the lump is cancerous and discharge her
D. Refer the patient for urgent mammography
E. Refer the patient for urgent ultrasound scan

24. ENDOCRINE DISEASE (4)

A 46-year-old woman attends a follow-up appointment at the endocrine surgery outpatient clinic. She had an operation for Cushing disease in the past. She complains that her skin is becoming darker and denies sun bed use or excess sunlight exposure.

What is the most likely diagnosis?

A. Acromegaly
B. Carcinoid syndrome
C. Conn syndrome
D. Hypoparathyroidism
E. Nelson syndrome

25. COLORECTAL OPERATIONS (1)

A 73-year-old woman presents to the surgical outpatient clinic with a 3-week history of rectal bleeding, a sensation of incomplete emptying despite defaecation and rectal discomfort. She is found to have a tumour 2 cm from the anal margin.

Which of the following would be the most appropriate operative intervention?

A. Abdominoperineal resection
B. Anterior resection
C. Hartmann procedure
D. Left hemicolectomy
E. Right hemicolectomy

26. CLASSIFICATION OF HERNIAS (1)

A 43-year-old woman presents to the GP with a lump in the right groin, which she says has been there on and off for a few months, but is now persistent. She has no other symptoms of note. On examination, there is a grape-sized lump below and lateral to the pubic tubercle. It is not tender and there is no cough impulse felt.

What is the most likely diagnosis?

A. Incarcerated femoral hernia
B. Incarcerated inguinal hernia
C. Obstructed femoral hernia
D. Strangulated femoral hernia
E. Strangulated inguinal hernia

27. SKIN LESIONS (4)

A 32-year-old man presents to the GP with multiple lesions on his trunk which have appeared over the last few months. Each lesion is raised, firm and rubbery, and causes a tingling sensation when touched.

Which of the following is the most likely diagnosis?

A. Ganglion
B. Granuloma annulare
C. Kaposi sarcoma

D. Neurofibroma

E. Sebaceous cyst

28. UPPER LIMB NERVE LESIONS (3)

An 82-year-old woman attends the emergency department following a fall. On examination, there is bruising over the left upper arm and the patient is unable to extend the metacarpals on the same side. There is loss of sensation over the lateral dorsal aspect of the hand.

Which nerve has most likely been affected?

A. Anterior interosseous nerve

B. Median nerve

C. Posterior interosseous nerve

D. Radial nerve

E. Upper brachial plexus

29. NECK LUMPS (4)

A 56-year-old woman presents with a lump on the left side of her neck which has been slowly enlarging over the last few months. On examination, there is a 2 cm firm, painless, mobile lump near the angle of the left jaw. She is still able to move her facial muscles.

What is the most likely diagnosis?

A. Chemodectoma

B. Pleomorphic adenoma

C. Salivary duct carcinoma

D. Salivary duct stone

E. Sternocleidomastoid tumour

30. EAR DISEASE (1)

A 46-year-old woman presents to the GP complaining of gradually progressive hearing loss, imbalance and tingling on the left side of her face. On examination, the patient admits that a vibrating tuning fork is louder when placed by the ear on the left side, rather than on the mastoid process.

Which of the following is the most likely cause of her symptoms?

A. Acoustic neuroma

B. Ménière disease

C. Otosclerosis

D. Perforated eardrum

E. Presbycusis

31. MANAGING UROLOGICAL DISEASE (2)

A 34-year-old man with a history of renal stones presents with a 3-hour history of right-sided loin pain. On examination, he looks unwell and his right kidney is palpable. The presence of a large stone is confirmed on X-ray. Blood results show a urea of 25 mmol/L and a creatinine of 400 μmol/L. On his previous admission last month, his urea and electrolytes were normal.

Which of the following would be indicated in the first instance?

A. Extracorporeal shock wave lithotripsy
B. Nephrectomy
C. Percutaneous nephrolithotomy
D. Percutaneous nephrostomy
E. Ureteroscopy

32. CHEST TRAUMA (4)

A 27-year-old man is brought into the emergency department following an assault. On arrival he has multiple bruises over the left side of his chest and upper abdomen. On examination, he has abdominal tenderness with guarding throughout. His observations include a heart rate of 132/min and blood pressure 86/42 mmHg. A chest X-ray shows a lower rib fracture and elevated diaphragm on the left.

Which of the following is the most likely cause of his symptoms?

A. Hepatic injury
B. Left-sided haemothorax
C. Left-sided pneumothorax
D. Ruptured diaphragm
E. Splenic injury

33. CONSENT

A 58-year-old man is admitted to hospital with a strangulated paraumbilical hernia that requires urgent operative intervention. He has a history of severe depression and is currently under Section for treatment of his mental condition. The patient does not consent to treatment even though he understands his condition, the benefits of having an operation and the potential outcomes of not having it.

Which is the most appropriate course of action?

A. Doctor can consent for the patient
B. Doctor can treat the patient under duty of care
C. Doctor can treat the patient under the Mental Health Act
D. Patient's refusal to treatment is valid and cannot be overridden
E. Patient's refusal to treatment is invalid and can be overridden

34. ORAL PATHOLOGY

A 71-year-old man presents to the GP with a painful, enlarging lump just in front of his right ear, which has been present for 2 months. He woke this morning to find that the right side of his face was drooping.

What is the most likely cause of his symptoms?

A. Acute bacterial sialothiasis
B. Parotitis
C. Pleomorphic adenoma
D. Salivary gland calculi
E. Salivary gland carcinoma

35. ABDOMINAL PAIN (12)

A 73-year-old woman presents to the emergency department with abdominal pain, vomiting and an inability to open her bowels. On examination, the abdomen is distended and the rectum is empty. The patient's husband tells you that she has lost a significant amount of weight over the last month and has been having blood in her stool.

Which of the following is the most likely cause of the presentation?

A. Colorectal malignancy
B. Constipation
C. Diverticulitis
D. Inguinal hernia
E. Ulcerative colitis

36. MANAGING BILIARY TRACT DISEASE (2)

A 40-year-old woman presents with intermittent episodes of severe right upper quadrant pain associated with meals. She is otherwise well and haemodynamically stable. Examination is unremarkable. .

Which of the following investigations would you perform in the first instance?

A. Abdominal ultrasound
B. Abdominal X-ray
C. ERCP
D. MRCP
E. Upper GI endoscopy

37. PAEDIATRIC ORTHOPAEDICS (4)

A 12-year-old boy presents to the emergency department with left-sided hip pain radiating to the knee. It started after he was running for a bus that morning. On examination, the boy is afebrile, overweight and the left leg is shortened and externally rotated.

Which of the following is the most likely cause of his symptoms?

A. Acute fracture of the hip
B. Perthes disease
C. Septic arthritis
D. Slipped upper femoral epiphysis
E. Spontaneous haemarthrosis

38. BACK PAIN (2)

A 53-year-old man presents to the emergency department in the middle of the night complaining of sudden-onset numbness and weakness below the waist. He has also had some urinary incontinence. On examination, his ankle reflexes are absent and he has marked weakness on both dorsal and plantar flexion of the feet. There is reduced anal tone on per rectum examination.

Which of the following is the most appropriate step?

A. Admit for urgent CT spine in the morning
B. Admit for urgent MRI spine in the morning
C. Obtain pelvic X-rays
D. Request urgent urology input
E. Transfer patient to a specialist spinal centre

39. UROLOGICAL CONDITIONS (1)

A 69-year-old man with poorly controlled insulin-dependent diabetes mellitus comes to see you in the urology outpatient department complaining of troublesome incontinence. He tells you he does not feel the urge to pass urine.

What is the most likely cause?

A. Atonic bladder
B. Benign prostatic hypertrophy
C. Bladder calculi
D. Detrusor instability
E. Urinary tract infection

40. GLASGOW COMA SCORE (2)

A 45-year-old man is brought into the emergency department following a fall from the balcony of his fourth floor flat. On arrival he makes no sound, does not open his eyes to pain and makes no motor response to any stimulus.

What is his Glasgow coma score?

A. 0
B. 1
C. 3
D. 6
E. 9

41. MANAGEMENT OF HERNIAS (1)

An 87-year-old woman with a history of chronic obstructive pulmonary disease with recurrent episodes of bronchitis comes to see you at the GP practice. She has noticed a lump in the lower abdomen when she stands. It does not cause her any concern but she just wanted to get it checked out.

On examination, she is obese and there is a soft, non-tender reducible mass in the lower abdomen. You note lower midline scarring from previous caesarean sections overlying the lump.

What would be the best course of management?

A. Conservative treatment unless symptoms change
B. Elective laparoscopic repair
C. Elective open repair
D. Emergency open repair
E. Prompt laparoscopic repair

42. INVESTIGATING VASCULAR DISEASE (2)

A 55-year-old man who has been a smoker for over 30 years has been referred to the surgical outpatient clinic with a 6-month history of severe calf pain on walking which is eased by rest. Blood tests requested by the GP are unremarkable.

Which of the following imaging investigations would you send him for?

A. CT scan
B. Digital subtraction angiography
C. Labelled white cell scan
D. MR angiogram
E. Ultrasound Doppler

43. MANAGING SKIN CONDITIONS (2)

A 42-year-old woman presents to the emergency department with swelling and redness in her left cheek and malaise which has been present for 1 day. On examination, the area of erythema is well demarcated and is hot to touch. Her observations include: heart rate 106/min, blood pressure 108/68 mmHg and temperature 38.6°C.

Which of the following is the best course of management?

A. 5-Fluorouracil
B. Analgesia
C. Intravenous antibiotics
D. Oral antibiotics
E. Surgical debridement

44. MANAGING ABDOMINAL PAIN (4)

A 68-year-old man is brought into the resuscitation room having been found collapsed outside a shop. On examination, he is pale, drowsy, and has a pulsatile mass in the abdomen. His observations include a heart rate of 126/min and a blood pressure of 86/38 mmHg.

Which of the following would be most appropriate?

A. Abdominal ultrasound
B. Abdominal X-ray

C. Aggressive fluid resuscitation
D. CT abdomen
E. Laparotomy

45. ACUTE LIMB ISCHAEMIA

A 64-year-old woman presents to the emergency department with an acutely painful left leg. She is complaining that it feels 'cold and numb'. There is no history of trauma and she has never had similar symptoms in the past.

Which of the following would you *not* expect to be found on examination?

A. A tender, pulsatile, expansile mass in the abdomen
B. Absent left leg pulses
C. ECG showing an irregular rhythm
D. Pan-systolic murmur on auscultation
E. Wet gangrene

46. HAND DISORDERS (2)

A 57-year-old man presents with a progressive deformity of his right hand which has been present for over a year. On examination, he has thickening over the palm with fixed contracture of the ring and little finger. He tells you that the deformity is limiting his day-to-day work as a computer programmer.

Which of the following management options would be recommended?

A. Conservative management
B. Physiotherapy
C. Splinting
D. Steroid injections
E. Surgery

47. THYROID DISEASE (4)

A 46-year-old woman attends her general practice complaining of low mood and tiredness. She has had this for a few months and has had to take time off work. On further questioning she admits to being constipated and to having gained 2 stone in weight over the previous month. On examination, no abnormality is apparent in the neck and no lymphadenopathy is palpable.

What is the most likely diagnosis?

A. Haemorrhage into a cyst
B. Hashimoto thyroiditis
C. Medullary carcinoma
D. Myxoedema coma
E. Primary myxoedema

48. PAEDIATRIC SURGERY (4)

A 3-year-old boy is brought to the GP practice by his mother. He has been complaining intermittently about abdominal pain. His mother feels that his abdomen is distended. On examination, there is a large mass on the left side of the abdomen which does not cross the midline.

What is the most likely diagnosis?

A. Hepatoblastoma
B. Lipoma
C. Nephroblastoma
D. Neuroblastoma
E. Polycystic kidney

49. MANAGING COMMON FRACTURES (2)

A 53-year-old woman has fallen onto her outstretched right hand, resulting in an undisplaced fracture of the distal radius and ulna. She was previously fit and well. She wants to know how long it will take for the fracture to heal.

How long would you expect this fracture to take to heal?

A. 1 week
B. 3 weeks
C. 6 weeks
D. 12 weeks
E. 16 weeks

50. STATISTICS (2)

Tented T waves on electrocardiograms are thought to reflect hyperkalaemia. A new proposed definition of tented T waves is 'a T wave that is taller than 2 large squares'. A study looking at the feasibility of this definition found 1000 ECGs: 200 with tented T waves (according to the proposed definitions) and 800 without. The study found that of the 200 people with ECGs with tented T waves, 100 had hyperkalaemia. Of the 800 people without tented T waves, a further 100 had hyperkalaemia.

What is the specificity of this definition of tented T waves with relation to hyperkalaemia?

A. 12.5%
B. 25.0%
C. 50.0%
D. 87.5%
E. 95.0%

Practice Paper 4: Answers

1. BONE PAIN (2)

D – Raised alkaline phosphatase and normal calcium

This patient has presented with features of Paget bone disease (also known as osteitis deformans). Paget disease is a disorder of bone remodelling, characterized by excessive bone reabsorption by osteoclasis, followed by a compensatory increase in bone formation by osteoblasts. This new bone, however, is structurally weaker and more vascular than normal bone, leading to deformity, increased susceptibility to fractures and high output cardiac failure. It most commonly affects people from the age of 50 upwards and is more common in males. Paget disease most commonly affects the skull, spine, pelvis and legs. The alkaline phosphatase is always raised. Calcium, phosphate, alanine transferase and parathyroid levels are normal, except in the setting of prolonged immobility, where hypercalcaemia may ensue. Characteristic appearances are found on X-ray; the bone cortex appears spongy, there is marked coarsening of the trabeculae and the whole bone is thickened. Treatment is largely with bisphosphonates, which inhibit bone reabsorption. Complications of Paget disease include pathological fractures, compression of cranial nerves within an enlarging skull, and the development of osteosarcomas.

Sir James Paget, English surgeon (1814–1899).

2. MANAGING DYSPHAGIA

C – Heller myotomy

This patient has presented with the symptoms and signs of oesophageal achalasia, a condition where there is failure of relaxation of the lower end of the oesophagus, due to a loss of ganglion cells in the myenteric plexus. It is generally a primary disorder but can also occur secondary to malignancy and Chagas disease. It typically presents between the ages of 20 and 40 years with an equal incidence in males and females. Surgical treatment involves incising the outer muscle layers of the lower oesophagus to the upper end of the stomach (Heller myotomy) often in combination with fundoplication of the stomach to prevent reflux. Medical treatments include calcium channel blockers (nifedipine) and the injection of botulinum toxin.

Ramstedt pyloromyotomy is a similar procedure performed for pyloric stenosis. Whipple procedure is used in resecting pancreatic carcinomas. Billroth I is a partial gastrectomy and Billroth II is partial gastrectomy with anastomosis of the stomach to the jejunum. These procedures have been used in the treatment of gastric ulcers and malignancies.

Ernst Heller, German surgeon (1877–1964).

3. BURNS (2)

C – 28%

Assessing the extent of burns is done quickly using Wallace's 'rule of nines'. The body is divided into units divisible by nine as follows:

Head + neck	→	9%	
Upper limb	→	9% each	
Anterior torso	→	18%	
Posterior torso	→	18%	
Lower limb	→	18% each	
Perineum	→	1%	(Total 100%)

In this example: front torso = 18%, right arm = 9%, left hand = 1%; giving a total of 28% burns.

4. FEMORAL NECK FRACTURES (1)

D – Reduction and internal fixation

The blood supply to the femoral head is three-fold: through the retinacular vessels at the base of the femoral neck (outside the capsule of the hip joint), through the intramedullary vessels, and through the ligamentum teres (which in the adult is usually negligible). Fractures can interrupt the blood supply, and a fracture that occurs within the joint capsule (intracapsular) disrupts the blood supply through both the retinacular and medullary vessels. An extracapsular fracture only disrupts the medullary blood supply. As a result, intracapsular femoral neck fractures carry a high risk of avascular necrosis of the femoral head. The treatment of such displaced fractures depends on the age of the patient. In older patients (over the age of 65) the femoral head would be removed and replaced with a prosthesis, either in the form of a hemiarthroplasty or a total hip replacement (depending on the fitness of the individual). In the younger patient, much is done to try to preserve the femoral head, and therefore a fracture in such a case would be reduced and fixed. One option is the use of cannulated screws, which are also used in treating undisplaced intracapsular fractures in the elderly. A fractured neck of femur in the young is considered an orthopaedic emergency, as delay in treatment increases the likelihood of developing avascular necrosis. Dynamic hip screws are used in treating extracapsular femoral neck fractures.

5. LOWER LIMB NERVE LESIONS (4)

B – Femoral nerve

The femoral nerve enters the thigh via the femoral triangle, where it lies lateral to the femoral artery. It can easily be damaged by penetrating wounds, hip dislocations or thigh haematomas. The femoral nerve supplies motor branches to the quadriceps, and sensory branches to the anterior thigh and medial calf (via the saphenous nerve). Femoral nerve palsies result in a loss of knee extension and loss of sensation over the anterior thigh and medial leg.

Femoral, from Latin *femur* = thigh.

6. LOCAL ANAESTHETIC AGENTS (1)

C – Lidocaine alone

A local anaesthetic is a drug which reversibly inhibits the propagation of nerve impulses. It acts by transiently altering the neurone membrane permeability to sodium ions.

Before suturing a finger, anaesthesia is produced by doing a ring block. This involves injection of 1–2 mL of local anaesthetic either side of the proximal phalanx at the level of the web space where the digital nerves run, producing anaesthesia along the entire length of the digit. Lidocaine is a quick-acting local anaesthetic and is appropriate for ring blocks. Adrenaline causes vasoconstriction and has the advantages of slowing systemic absorption and prolonging duration of action of local anaesthetics. However, local anaesthetics containing adrenaline must *never* be used near end arteries (e.g. digits, nose and penis) as there is a risk of ischaemic necrosis.

The maximum dose of lidocaine is 3 mg/kg (or 7 mg/kg if given with adrenaline).

Lidocaine/prilocaine mixture can be given as a topical emulsion preparation to children before inserting a cannula or taking bloods. It is marketed under the trade name EMLA (eutetic mixture of local anaesthetic) and the emulsion is left on for 30–60 minutes to allow full dermal anaesthesia to take place. A 'eutetic' mixture is one that contains equal amounts of each ingredient. For example, EMLA contains 2.5% each of lidocaine and prilocaine. Other examples of topical local anaesthetics include Instillagel™ (lidocaine) used for urethral catheterization, and Xylocaine™ (lidocaine) spray given before upper gastrointestinal endoscopies. Amethocaine eye drops are used for conjunctival anaesthesia. Amethocaine is also available as a cream (Amitop™) and its onset of action of dermal anaesthesia is more rapid than EMLA.

Cocaine was the first compound to be used as a local anaesthetic. Its anaesthetic properties were discovered accidentally by Sigmund Freud (Austrian neurologist, psychiatrist and frequent cocaine user).

Cocaine has since been used in ophthalmic and nasal operations. Side effects of cocaine include intense vasoconstriction and cardiotoxicity, so it has now largely been replaced by benzocaine and proxymetacaine for ENT use.

7. X-RAY APPEARANCES OF GASTROINTESTINAL DISEASE

C – Diverticular outpouchings

This patient has presented with the symptoms of diverticular disease. Diverticula are caused by high intraluminal pressures within the colon, usually secondary to constipation, leading to the herniation of mucosa through weak points in the bowel wall (these being at the site of entry of blood vessels). Barium enema is a radiological technique in which contrast is used to assess the anatomy of the rectum and colon, and can be used to confirm the presence of diverticula (seen as outpouchings of contrast). An apple-core lesion is an annular constriction of the colon typical of colonic cancer. Barium enemas have in the past been used to confirm the diagnosis of appendicitis as an inflamed appendix that does not fill with barium. Thumb printing of the colon is seen in attacks of ischaemic colitis and represents areas of mucosal and submucosal haemorrhage and oedema.

8. ABDOMINAL PAIN (10)

B – Gastric cancer

Gastric cancer is the second most common cancer worldwide and is most common in the Japanese, Chinese and Russian populations. Its peak incidence is between the ages of 50 and 70, and men are more commonly affected than women. Presenting symptoms may be quite vague in the early stages and include epigastric pain, early satiety, vomiting, anorexia and weight loss. As a result, gastric cancers are often diagnosed late and have a poor prognosis (5-year survival of around 20%). The majority (95%) of gastric cancers are adenocarcinomas. Risk factors include *Helicobacter pylori* infection, smoking, and eating pickled and smoked foods. Patients with a history of chronic peptic ulceration, pernicious anaemia, Menetrier disease, and those who have had a previous gastrectomy are at greater risk of developing gastric carcinoma. External manifestations of metastasis include left-sided supraclavicular lymphadenopathy (Virchow node) and umbilical lumps (Sister Joseph's nodules). Transcoelomic spread of gastric cancer to the ovaries is known as Krukenberg tumours.

Pernicious anaemia is a megaloblastic anaemia caused by autoantibodies to gastric parietal cells, resulting in impaired absorption of vitamin B_{12} secondary to a lack of intrinsic factor. Damage to parietal cells results in anaemia and atrophic gastritis, secondary to achlorhydria.

Menetrier disease is a rare condition usually affecting young to middle-aged men. It is characterized by hyperplasia of mucus-producing cells within the stomach resulting in reduced acid secretion and a protein-losing enteropathy. Symptoms include epigastric pain, weight loss and peripheral oedema secondary to hypoalbuminaemia. There is a 10% risk of gastric carcinoma, so regular endoscopic surveillance is warranted.

Rudolf Ludwig Karl Virchow, German pathologist (1821–1901).

Friedrich Ernst Krukenberg, German gynaecologist (1871–1946).

9. DYSPHAGIA (4)

D – Pseudobulbar palsy

A pseudobulbar palsy is the result of a bilateral upper motor neurone lesion affecting the 9th to 12th cranial nerves inclusively. The lesion arises within the corticobulbar pathways or pyramidal tract. Causes include motor neurone disease, multiple sclerosis and brain stem tumours. Other signs include those of an upper motor neurone lesion in the limbs (spasticity, hyperreflexia, weakness without muscle wasting). By contrast, a *bulbar palsy* is caused by a bilateral lower motor neurone lesion of the 9th to 12th cranial nerves inclusively. It may also present with dysphagia and dysarthria. Other features include a wasted fasciculating tongue, drooling and an absent gag reflex. General features of a lower motor neurone lesion include hypotonicity, hyporeflexia and muscular fasciculations. The lesion in bulbar palsy may arise within the medulla, or from outside the brain stem. Causes include motor neurone disease, Guillain-Barré syndrome and myasthenia gravis.

Scleroderma is a chronic autoimmune condition of unknown cause, characterized by thickening of the skin and other organs. The condition may be localized, or diffuse (systemic sclerosis). Characteristic features are described by the CREST syndrome (Calcinosis, Raynaud's, oEsophageal dysmotility, Sclerodactyly and Telangiectasia). *Paralysis of the vocal cords* presents with hoarseness of the voice and dysphagia with regurgitation. Causes include neurological conditions, e.g. following cerebrovascular accident, tumours and tetanus. Bilateral vocal cord paralysis would result in respiratory distress and arrest. The vocal cords can be visualized and assessed by laryngoscopy.

10. MANAGING ENDOCRINE DISEASE (1)

A – Intravenous thyroxine

This patient has presented in a myxoedema coma, a medical emergency with a mortality of up to 50%. It is a severe, decompensated form of hypothyroidism with a marked reduction in free thyroxine. Myxoedema coma is four times more common in women and its incidence increases after the age of 50. Myxoedema coma is more common in those with undiagnosed/untreated hypothyroidism and following thyroid surgery. It may also be precipitated by cold, infections, trauma and drugs such as amiodarone. Physical findings are those of severe hypothyroidism, namely hypothermia, hypotensive shock, non-pitting oedema, lethargy and reduced consciousness. Treatment must be aggressive and take place in an intensive care setting. Intravenous thyroxine is necessary, as is the rapid and adequate administration of treatment such as gentle re-warming and treatment of associated problems such as infection and hyponatraemia. Intubation and mechanical ventilation and cardiac monitoring may also be required.

Both propranolol and propylthiouracil are used in the treatment of a thyroid storm – a life-threatening emergency caused by excessive thyroid hormones. It presents with clinically opposite features including hyperthermia, hypertension, tachycardia, weight loss and altered behaviour. Treatment in both cases must not be delayed until blood results are available and should be based initially on clinical findings due to the high mortality.

11. JAUNDICE (4)

A – Alcoholic liver disease

Hepatitis is the name given to inflammation of the liver, regardless of the aetiology. Causes include infections (viral hepatitis), drugs (e.g. isoniazid), alcohol, abnormal metabolism (haemochromatosis) and autoimmune conditions. Hepatic damage caused by alcohol occurs in three stages: the first is the development of a fatty liver (reversible); the second an alcohol-induced hepatitis (partially reversible); and the third is cirrhosis – end-stage, irreversible liver damage. Symptoms of alcoholic liver disease may be very vague in the initial stages, including nausea and right upper quadrant pain. Jaundice, encephalopathy, ascites and caput medusa (dilated peri-umbilical veins) are signs of late irreversible disease. Around 10% of those with cirrhosis develop hepatocellular carcinoma. Alcohol-induced cirrhosis may be an indication for a liver transplant.

Hepatitis A is caused by an RNA virus which is spread by the faeco-oral route and is the most common cause of hepatitis worldwide. It is an acute condition causing gastrointestinal disturbance and jaundice. Treatment is supportive and the condition is largely self-limiting. *Hepatitis B* is a DNA virus that is spread by inoculation of bodily fluids. It causes an acute hepatitis which may become a chronic condition in some and result in liver cirrhosis. *Autoimmune hepatitis* is a condition of unknown cause. It is rare and most commonly affects young to middle-aged women. It is associated with other autoimmune conditions. Treatment is with immunosuppressants but the disease can progress to cirrhosis. *Reye syndrome* is characterized by encephalopathy and the presence of a fatty liver. It is associated with aspirin use in children.

12. ABNORMAL GLUCOSE METABOLISM

B – Increased C-peptide levels

This patient has presented with symptoms of hypoglycaemia, caused by an insulinoma. An insulinoma is a neuroendocrine tumour of the pancreatic beta cells resulting in autonomic insulin production leading to symptomatic hypoglycaemia. Insulinomas are characterized by Whipple's triad: episodic hypoglycaemia + central nervous system dysfunction (anxiety, confusion) + symptomatic relief by the administration of glucose. Blood results will show reduced blood glucose levels, elevated insulin levels (despite hypoglycaemia), elevated pro-insulin levels and elevated C-peptide levels. C-peptide is the by product of the cleavage of pro-insulin into insulin and can be used to differentiate cases of factitious hyperinsulinaemia, as in exogenous insulin administration, where C-peptide levels will not be elevated. Insulinomas are largely benign (90%) and may be part of the MEN I syndrome. Treatment is by excision of the tumour. Insulinomas are the most common type of pancreatic endocrine tumours. Glucagon increases blood glucose and somatostatin inhibits insulin production, therefore glucagonomas and somatostatinomas present with the features of hyperglycaemia.

13. PENILE CONDITIONS (2)

D – Referral to a specialist for corrective surgery

This boy has hypospadias, a condition in which there is incomplete tubularization of the urethra in the embryo, resulting in the urethral meatus being present below its normal opening at the glans. The meatus can be found anywhere from the under-surface of the glans to the perineum. Hypospadias occurs in up to 1 in 250 of male births. Problems include concern about cosmetic appearance, difficulty urinating and deformity on erection affecting sexual intercourse. Surgical correction is indicated if symptoms occur.

Hypospadias, from Greek *hupo* = under + *spas* = fissure/crack.

14. PAEDIATRIC SURGERY INVESTIGATION

C – Rectal biopsy

This child presented with signs of large bowel obstruction, as indicated by the failure of meconium passage. The most common cause for obstruction in the neonatal period is Hirschsprung disease – a congenital absence of ganglion cells from the myenteric plexus of the large bowel, resulting in a narrowed, contracted segment. The abnormally innervated bowel extends proximally from the rectum for a variable distance. Ten percent of cases affect the whole colon. It occurs in approximately 1/5000 births and is three times more common in males. Hirschsprung disease often presents in neonates with abdominal distension and bile-stained vomiting. Rectal examination shows a narrowed segment, and removal of the examining finger is often followed by a gush of stools and flatus. Less severe cases can present in later life with chronic constipation, abdominal distension, megacolon and occasionally offensive overflow diarrhoea. A definitive diagnosis is made by rectal biopsy which shows absent ganglion cells in the submucosa, with an increase in acetylcholinesterase cells in the muscularis mucosae. A barium enema will confirm the presence of a contracted rectum. Abdominal X-ray will confirm the diagnosis of obstruction but not the cause. Rectal examination may relieve obstruction temporarily by allowing the passage of meconium. Treatment of Hirschsprung disease involves an initial defunctioning colostomy to relieve the obstruction, followed by either excision or bypass of the affected segment of bowel.

Harald Hirschsprung, Danish paediatrician (1830–1916).

15. EPONYMOUS FRACTURES (1)

D – Monteggia fracture

A Monteggia fracture dislocation is caused by a fall with forced pronation of the forearm. It consists of a proximal ulna fracture with associated dislocation of the radial head. A Galeazzi fracture dislocation is a fracture of the radial shaft, at the junction of its middle and lower thirds, with dislocation of the distal ulna. If you see a forearm fracture on an X-ray, you should always look for an associated dislocation.

Giovanni Monteggia, Italian surgeon (1762–1815).

Ricardo Galeazzi, Italian surgeon (1866–1952).

16. ABDOMINAL PAIN (11)

A – Adhesions

This patient has presented with bowel obstruction. The typical symptoms of bowel obstruction are abdominal pain, distension, vomiting and absolute constipation (not passing faeces or wind). The clinical picture is dependent upon the site of obstruction: small bowel obstruction presents initially with central colicky abdominal pain, distension and vomiting; large bowel obstruction presents with lower abdominal pain, distension and constipation. Vomiting is usually a late sign in large bowel obstruction and tends to be faeculent. Obstruction may be mechanical or functional, where there is a reduction in normal peristaltic activity of the bowel. The most common causes of small bowel obstruction are adhesions and hernias. Common causes of large bowel obstruction are faecal impaction, hernias and tumours. Paralytic ileus commonly follows gastrointestinal surgery where there is excessive handling of bowel, and can be caused by electrolyte disturbances. Gallstones can cause obstruction if they erode through the gallbladder and into the duodenum, subsequently lodging distally at the ileocaecal junction (gallstone ileus). Abdominal X-ray may show air in the biliary tree or a stone at the ileocaecal junction, together with small bowel obstruction.

17. ANORECTAL DISEASE (3)

E – Proctalgia fugax

Proctalgia fugax is a benign condition that tends to affect young, anxious men. It is characterized by brief attacks of rectal pain which usually occur at night and are unrelated to defaecation. Management involves reassurance, analgesia and topical smooth muscle relaxants (e.g. GTN cream).

Proctalgia fugax, from Greek *proktos* = anus + *algos* = pain + *fugax* = fleeting.

18. ANATOMY OF HERNIAS (2)

E – Pantaloon

A pantaloon hernia is a type of direct inguinal hernia where the hernia sac straddles the inferior epigastric vessels. Normally, a direct inguinal hernia passes medial to the inferior epigastric vessels, whereas an indirect hernia lies lateral to these.

For a description of the other listed hernias, please see the question 'Anatomy of hernias (3)'.

19. AIRWAY MANAGEMENT (1)

A – Endotracheal intubation

Airway management in the trauma patient is dependent on the level of consciousness of the patient and the injuries sustained. A patient who is fully alert and talking is maintaining the airway and therefore supplemental oxygen via face mask is all that is required. With impaired consciousness, an oropharyngeal or nasopharyngeal airway would be required as assistance, depending on which is the better tolerated. A more conscious patient would not be able to tolerate an oropharyngeal airway. Any patient who is unconscious, and therefore unable to protect their airway, needs a definitive airway, i.e. endotracheal intubation. The jaw thrust can be performed in the immobilized patient to assist in opening the airway, but never hyperextend the neck as this can damage the cervical spine. There are certain situations where intubation may be considered early, such as in smoke inhalation or those at risk of respiratory arrest. There may be situations in which endotracheal intubation is not possible due to complete occlusion of the upper airway, e.g. severe facial injuries. In this situation, a needle cricothyroidotomy provides a temporary means of ventilation until a formal tracheostomy can be performed in theatre.

20. GROIN LUMPS (4)

D – Saphena varix

A saphena varix is a dilatation of the long saphenous vein that occurs due to valvular incompetence at the saphenofemoral junction (which is an inch below and lateral to the pubic tubercle, just medial to the femoral pulse). A saphena varix often has a bluish tinge, is soft and compressible, disappears on lying down, has a cough impulse and exhibits a fluid thrill when the long saphenous vein is tapped distally (Schwartz test). It is often associated with varicosities elsewhere in the saphenous system.

A psoas abscess is a recognized complication of tuberculosis following the development of a paraspinal abscess (Pott's disease). If this abscess tracks down the psoas muscle towards the groin, an inguinal psoas abscess can arise. A psoas abscess is usually fluctuant, painless and not warm (hence it is given the term 'cold abscess' which is characteristic of tuberculosis infection). The diagnosis of a psoas abscess is best made by MRI.

Percival Pott, British surgeon (1714–1788).

21. INVESTIGATING ABDOMINAL PAIN (4)

E – Urine pregnancy test

In any female of child-bearing age presenting with an acute abdomen a urine pregnancy test must be done in the first instance, in view of an ectopic pregnancy being the potential cause. An ectopic pregnancy is one that implants outside the uterus, most commonly in the fallopian tubes. It occurs in up to 1% of pregnancies and is associated with a history of pelvic inflammatory disease, intra-uterine contraceptive devices, progesterone-only pills, previous tubal surgery and previous ectopic pregnancy.

Ectopic pregnancy can present with amenorrhoea, abnormal vaginal spotting or bleeding, or vague abdominal pain. Rupture of an ectopic pregnancy causes acute abdominal pain. Clinically there may be localized guarding or generalized peritonitis with a rigid abdomen. Blood loss results in shock. Urgent resuscitation is required in these cases with either laparotomy or laparoscopy to remove the ectopic pregnancy. In early pregnancy, abdominal ultrasound may not be sensitive enough to detect the conceptus; a transvaginal scan is more sensitive. If the diagnosis is in doubt, serial measurements of serum beta-hCG can be performed. In normal pregnancies this will double every 2 days, but in an ectopic pregnancy the doubling time will be prolonged.

Ectopic, from Greek *ek* = away from + *topos* = place, i.e. in the wrong place.

22. KNEE CONDITIONS (2)

D – Osteochondritis dissecans

Osteochondritis dissecans is characterized by local ischaemic necrosis of a segment of the articular surface of a bone and its overlying cartilage. There is eventual separation of the fragment which results in an intra-articular loose body. The knee is the most common site for osteochondritis dissecans, especially the medial condyle of the femur. If the intra-articular loose body becomes trapped in the joint, the patient experiences sudden 'locking' of the knee associated with severe pain and swelling (as in this scenario). Loose bodies in the knee can often be seen by radiography and are usually found in the suprapatellar pouch (they are occasionally palpable here). Management is by removal of the loose body using arthroscopy.

In *chondromalacia patellae* the cartilage of the articular surface of the patella becomes roughened. The pain is caused by friction between the damaged area and the femoral condyle. Chondromalacia patellae presents in teenage girls with an aching pain behind the kneecap which is exacerbated by climbing and descending stairs. X-rays show no abnormality.

The *pre-patellar bursa* lies in front of the lower half of the patella and the upper part of the patellar tendon. Repeated friction of the bursa, usually in those who kneel, results in pain and swelling of the bursa. This is known as prepatellar bursitis, or housemaid's knee. Management can either be by aspiration (although recurrence may occur) or excision of the offending bursa.

Chondromalacia, from Greek *khondros* = cartilage + *malakos* = soft.

Dissecans, from Latin *dissecare* = to separate.

23. INVESTIGATING BREAST DISEASE (1)

E – Refer the patient for urgent ultrasound scan

Although most breast cancers occur in women over the age of 40 (with incidence markedly increasing after the age of 50), younger women tend to develop the most aggressive forms of breast cancer, accounting for the lower survival rates. Therefore all breast lumps must be investigated or at least referred to the breast clinic for assessment. Mammography is the first-line imaging choice in the older woman (over 40 years); however, the increased breast density in younger patients makes ultrasound investigation more sensitive. Most malignant breast lumps are painless, so this is not a reliable indicator of serious pathology; neither is the size of the lump. In this age group the most likely cause of a breast lump is a benign fibroadenoma.

24. ENDOCRINE DISEASE (4)

E – Nelson syndrome

This woman has been treated for Cushing disease in the past. Cushing disease describes the presence of an ACTH-secreting tumour in the pituitary that results in excess cortisol and features of Cushing syndrome. The treatment of Cushing disease is usually by removal of the primary tumour. However, in occasional cases where the tumour is occult, bilateral adrenalectomy is performed to eliminate the production of cortisol. The lack of cortisol's negative feedback on the pituitary allows the pre-existing pituitary ACTH tumour to grow rapidly. This process is known as Nelson syndrome and occurs after 20% of bilateral adrenalectomies. The excess ACTH of Nelson syndrome results in skin hyperpigmentation via the secretion of melanocyte stimulating hormone.

Nelson D, Meakin J, Thorn G. ACTH-producing pituitary tumors following adrenalectomy for Cushing syndrome. *Ann Intern Med* 1960;52:560–9.

25. COLORECTAL OPERATIONS (1)

A – Abdominoperineal resection

Rectal tumours account for a third of cases of colorectal cancers, and the majority of these are adenocarcinomas. They most commonly occur in the seventh decade, especially in men and in Western populations. The overall lifetime risk of developing colorectal cancer is around 6% and the majority of cases have no obvious identifiable risk factors. Specific risk factors include familial adenomatous polyposis, hereditary non-polyposis colorectal cancer, a family history and inflammatory bowel disease. The treatment of colorectal cancers is dependent on the site of the tumour.

Abdominoperineal resections are performed when the tumour lies in the distal third of the rectum (within 8 cm of the anus). In this procedure, both abdominal and perineal incisions are made and the anus, rectum and part of the sigmoid colon removed with the remaining sigmoid colon being brought out as a permanent colostomy. Anterior resections are used in tumours of the proximal two-thirds of the rectum. Following tumour removal, an anastomosis is made between the sigmoid and the lower rectum. Right hemicolectomy is performed for non-obstructing tumours of the right side of the colon. This involves removal of the distal ileum, ascending colon and the proximal portion of the transverse colon. The right hemicolectomy may be extended if the tumour is situated in the transverse colon or at the hepatic flexure. Left hemicolectomy is used for non-obstructing tumours of the descending colon and splenic flexure.

26. CLASSIFICATION OF HERNIAS (1)

A – Incarcerated femoral hernia

A hernia is the abnormal protrusion of the whole, or part, of a viscus through its containing walls. A femoral hernia is the protrusion of contents, i.e. extraperitoneal fat, omentum or bowel, into the potential space of the femoral canal. Femoral hernias are three times more common in women than men and more commonly occur on the right side. They are differentiated from inguinal hernias in that they lie below and lateral to the pubic tubercle. Inguinal hernias are caused by weakness in the abdominal wall at the entrance to the inguinal canal. They may be indirect (75%), passing through the internal inguinal ring and down the inguinal canal, or direct, passing through the posterior wall of the canal but not down the canal. Inguinal hernias are found above and medial to the pubic tubercle. The contents of a hernia may be returned to the abdominal cavity either spontaneously or with direct pressure, and this is described as a reducible hernia. There will be a cough impulse on examination. Hernias which cannot be returned to the abdominal cavity are described as irreducible or incarcerated. There will be no cough impulse on examination. Both reducible and incarcerated hernias are typically painless.

A strangulated hernia is one in which the blood supply to the contents is cut off; in other words where an irreducible hernia develops oedema and venous congestion, causing pressure on the arterial supply. The area subsequently becomes ischaemic and then gangrenous. Strangulation is common in femoral hernias due to the narrow neck of the femoral canal. Obstruction of bowel within the hernia sac presents with the typical features of vomiting, colicky abdominal pain, distension and absolute constipation, and may be associated with strangulation of bowel. If untreated, perforation and peritonitis occur. Strangulated and obstructed hernias are surgical emergencies.

Hernia, from Greek *hernias* = to sprout forth.

27. SKIN LESIONS (4)

D – Neurofibroma
Neurofibromas are benign neoplasms of the nerve sheaths of central or peripheral nerves that feel firm and rubbery. Neurofibromas may be single or multiple, as in neurofibromatosis. Neurofibromatosis (NF) is an autosomal dominant disorder characterized by multiple neurofibromas, coffee-coloured macules (café-au-lait patches) and axillary freckling with a risk of developing central nervous system tumours (acoustic neuroma, optic glioma, meningioma), iris fibromas (Lisch nodules) and phaeochromocytomas. There are two types of neurofibromatosis (NF): NF1 (von Recklinghausen disease) is the 'peripheral' form which displays the cutaneous manifestations; and NF2 is the 'central' form with bilateral central nervous systems tumours and very few cutaneous features.

Friedrich von Recklinghausen, German pathologist (1833–1910).

28. UPPER LIMB NERVE LESIONS (3)

D – Radial nerve
The radial nerve runs in close proximity to the shaft of the humerus in the spiral groove. Common causes of radial nerve palsies include humeral shaft fractures (as in this scenario, in which case patients also suffer bruising to the upper arm), compression of the nerve in the arm with prolonged

use of ill-fitting crutches and elbow dislocations or Monteggia fractures. Damage to the radial nerve is also seen in people who fall asleep with their arm hanging over the back of a chair ('Saturday night palsy'). The radial nerve supplies the extensors to the forearm and wrist, and a radial nerve palsy results in an inability to extend the wrist or metacarpophalangeal joints (wrist drop), forearm extensor wasting and a loss of sensation in the anatomical snuffbox. The anatomical snuffbox is the name given to the triangular region on the radial dorsal aspect of the hand at the level of the carpal bones. It is so called because it was the surface used since the 16th century for placing and snorting 'snuff' (powdered tobacco).

The *posterior interosseous nerve* is a branch of the radial nerve that runs deep in the forearm to supply the wrist and finger extensors except the extensor carpi radialis longus (which is innervated by a proximal branch from the radial nerve). The posterior interosseous nerve can be damaged in forearm fractures and results in an inability to extend the fingers and a weak wrist drop. The wrist drop is only slight as the extensor carpi radialis longus muscle still provides some wrist extension. There is no sensory loss with these nerve lesions.

The *anterior interosseous nerve* is a motor branch of the median nerve in the forearm. Lesions of this nerve are rare and usually arise from deep lacerations to the forearm. The anterior interosseous nerve provides motor fibres to flexor pollicis longus, the medial part of flexor digitorum profundus and pronator quadratus. Patients have a weakness in the thumb and index finger characterized by a deformity in the pinch mechanism between the thumb and index finger.

29. NECK LUMPS (4)

B – Pleomorphic adenoma

A hard, painless mobile lump near the angle of the jaw in a woman of this age, with no evidence of facial nerve involvement, is likely to be a pleomorphic adenoma. The pleomorphic adenoma is the most common benign tumour of the salivary glands. It is most common in the 40s to 50s and the only known risk factor is exposure to radiation. The facial nerve is characteristically not involved (if it were, this feature would imply malignancy). Treatment is by excision of the tumour, which has a good prognosis.

30. EAR DISEASE (1)

A – Acoustic neuroma

Hearing loss may be conductive or sensorineural in origin. In conductive deafness, sound is not transmitted to the inner ear, the abnormality being in the external or middle ear. Sensorineural deafness is a result of pathology within the cochlea or the vestibulocochlear nerve and/or its transmission of signals to the brain. Conductive and sensorineural deafness may be differentiated by using a tuning fork. The examining doctor in this scenario has performed the Rinne test. In this investigation a vibrating tuning fork of 512 Hz (an octave above 'middle C') is placed initially on the mastoid process (bone conduction), and then next to the ear (air conduction). The patient is then asked which sound was loudest. In the normal ear, air conduction (AC) is better than bone conduction (BC) – this is known as a positive Rinne test. In the woman in this scenario, AC is better than BC – this positive Rinne test with left-sided deafness is associated with a sensorineural hearing loss. The second clinical test often used when examining hearing is the Weber test. In this test a vibrating 512 Hz tuning fork is placed in the middle of the patient's forehead. The patient is asked to report in which ear the sound is loudest. In conductive deafness, the sound is heard louder in the deafer ear. In sensorineural deafness the sound is heard louder in the better ear.

An acoustic neuroma is a benign tumour of the Schwann cells of the vestibulocochlear nerve, more predominant in women between the fourth and seventh decade. Its cause is unknown but it develops bilaterally in those with type 2 neurofibromatosis. Features of an acoustic neuroma include hearing loss, tinnitus, imbalance, facial sensory disturbance (due to the close proximity to the trigeminal nerve) and weakness of the facial muscles on the affected side (facial nerve compression). Symptoms of raised intracranial pressure (headache, visual loss) occur if the neuroma is large. Acoustic neuromas are best seen on MRI. Treatment may be observation (if the neuroma is small) or surgical removal.

Otosclerosis is a conductive form of deafness caused by the overgrowth and sclerosis of the temporal bone resulting in a 'fixed' stapes. It is a progressive condition seen most commonly in Caucasian females, and goes on to affect both ears. It is inherited as an autosomal dominant condition, but has variable penetrance. A common symptom is paracusis (hearing is better when there is background noise). Symptoms are aggravated by pregnancy. Treatment is by stapedectomy and stapes implant. *Presbycusis* is the name given to age related deafness. It is sensorineural in origin, caused by the degeneration of the nerve cells within the inner ear. It is the most common form of deafness with progressive age and is bilateral. The onset of presbycusis may be hastened by certain drugs (e.g. aspirin) and repetitive noise trauma.

Ménières disease is a condition of unknown aetiology affecting the labyrinth of the inner ear. Symptoms are usually intermittent and include vertigo, tinnitus and difficulty hearing low frequency sounds. There is an association with viral infections. Treatment is largely symptomatic and includes antihistamines and prochlorperazine. A *perforated eardrum* can occur following trauma, infection and sudden loud noises. The level of deafness is dependent on the size of the perforation, which usually heals itself within 8 weeks. Rarely a tympanoplasty may be required.

Otosclerosis, from Greek *oto* = ear + *skleros* = hard; 'hardening of the ear'.
Acoustic, from Greek *akoustikos* = to hear.
Prosper Ménière, French physician (1799–1862).
Heinrich Adolf Rinne, German ENT surgeon (1819–1868).
Ernst Heinrich Weber, German physiologist and psychologist (1795–1878).

31. MANAGING UROLOGICAL DISEASE (2)

D – Percutaneous nephrostomy

This patient has presented with acute renal failure secondary to urinary tract obstruction by a renal calculus. This is a urological emergency and must be managed immediately to prevent irreversible damage to the kidneys. A percutaneous nephrostomy, which is the insertion of a catheter into the renal pelvis through the skin, creates a temporary diversion of urine, reducing the back-pressure on the kidney and giving time for formal removal of the stone. Percutaneous nephrostomies are performed under radiological guidance and local anaesthesia. Other indications for percutaneous nephrostomy include the diversion of urine following damage to the ureters, obstruction secondary to pregnancy, and to allow the drainage of a perinephric abscess. Insertion is contraindicated in those with a bleeding diathesis. Complications of percutaneous nephrostomy include haemorrhage, sepsis and damage to surrounding organs (e.g. pneumothorax).

Extracorporeal shock wave lithotripsy uses sound waves, which penetrate the skin, to break large renal calculi into smaller fragments that can be passed more easily by the patient. It can be performed easily as an outpatient procedure, under local anaesthesia. Percutaneous nephrolithotomy allows the removal of stones from the upper ureter and kidney without having to perform an open procedure. A guide wire is inserted under radiological guidance and a tract is made through which the stone can be removed. Ureteroscopy is a procedure in which a fine bore endoscope is inserted into the ureter via the urethra. It is performed under general or epidural anaesthesia. Indications include removal of ureteric stones, insertion of a ureteric stent and dilatation of strictures. Nephrectomy is the surgical removal of the kidney. It may be done as an open or laparoscopic procedure. Indications for nephrectomy include localized renal cell carcinoma and an irreversibly malfunctioning kidney.

32. CHEST TRAUMA (4)

E – Splenic injury

The spleen is the most vascular organ in the body, containing up to one unit of blood at any time. Splenic injuries are therefore potentially life threatening. The spleen is the most commonly injured organ in cases of thoraco-abdominal trauma, particularly with blunt injuries. It is commonly associated with lower left-sided rib fractures. The presentation of splenic trauma depends on the extent of damage and may vary from vague upper left-sided abdominal pain (in cases of a subcapsular haematoma) to shock and peritonitis with splenic rupture. Up to 50% of patients with a ruptured spleen have other intraperitoneal injuries. The management of splenic trauma depends upon the stability of the patient. Unstable patients require resuscitation and transfer to theatre. The most suitable imaging technique in the stable patient would be a CT scan which would not only confirm the diagnosis but assess the severity of damage. The triad of an elevated left hemidiaphragm, left lower lobe atelectasis and pleural effusion in splenic rupture is rarely seen on chest X-ray; however any patient with hemidiaphragm elevation should be considered to have a splenic injury unless otherwise proved.

Splenic injuries may be graded as follows:

1. Minor subcapsular tear or haematoma
2. Parenchymal injury not extending to the hilum
3. Parenchymal injury involving the hilum and vessels
4. Shattered spleen

Grade 1 and 2 splenic injuries may be treated conservatively on a watch and wait basis. Grade 3 injuries are treated with splenic repair and grade 4 injuries with splenectomy. Asplenic patients are at risk of thrombosis and serious infections by encapsulated bacteria (*Pneumococcus* and *Meningococcus*). Lifelong prophylaxis with penicillin is therefore required.

Rupture of the diaphragm is usually the result of blunt abdominal trauma and commonly occurs with splenic injury. The majority of diaphragmatic ruptures occur on the left (due to the protection by the liver on the right) and posteriorly (a congenitally weaker area). Large lacerations result in the herniation of abdominal contents into the thorax causing respiratory distress. On examination there will be reduced air entry on the affected side and paradoxical movement of the abdomen. Bowel sounds may be heard in the chest. Treatment is by surgical repair.

33. CONSENT

D – Patient's refusal to treatment is valid and cannot be overridden

This patient understands the risks and benefits of surgery and, as such, can be deemed to have the capacity to make an informed decision, irrespective of his chronic mental health problems. The Mental Health Act does not allow for treatment of any medical condition other than a psychiatric disorder. Similarly, no adult can 'consent' for another adult. The patient's refusal to treatment is therefore valid and the doctor cannot override it.

34. ORAL PATHOLOGY

E – Salivary gland carcinoma

Salivary gland carcinomas are rare aggressive tumours most commonly occurring in the parotid gland. They are three times more common in men and rarely occur in the under 50s. Patients present with a rapidly growing mass, and there may be features of infiltration, e.g. facial nerve involvement and regional palpable lymph nodes. Treatment involves parotidectomy with radiotherapy. Prognosis is poor.

A *pleomorphic adenoma* is a benign tumour of the salivary glands, more commonly affecting the parotid gland. The name arises from the typical variable appearance of the tumours with light microscopy. Presentation is with a slow growing, firm, painless mass. Treatment is by surgical resection. Salivary tumours should be investigated with imaging and biopsy to determine whether they are malignant or benign. *Salivary gland calculi* are calcium stones that cause obstruction of the salivary ducts leading to intense pain and swelling of the affected gland while eating. The symptoms resolve within an hour or two. The submandibular gland duct (of Wharton) is the most common site. Diagnosis is by injecting a dye into the duct system (sialography), and treatment is by removing the stone. *Acute bacterial sialothiasis* is the result of superimposed bacterial infection within an obstructed salivary duct causing acute inflammation, pain and abscess formation. Intravenous antibiotics are required. Mumps is caused by a RNA paramyxovirus and causes painful enlargement of the salivary glands. It typically affects the parotid gland (parotitis), is largely bilateral and most commonly affects children. Treatment is symptomatic.

35. ABDOMINAL PAIN (12)

A – Colorectal malignancy

This patient has presented with the signs and symptoms of large bowel obstruction. Common causes in this age group include tumours, hernias, faecal impaction, volvulus and stricture formation following repeated episodes of diverticulitis. The history of weight loss and rectal bleeding would suggest a diagnosis of colorectal carcinoma. Colorectal cancer is the second most common cancer causing death in the UK. The term encompasses both cancers of the colon (60%) and rectum (40%), although in up to 5% of patients multiple sites are affected. The majority of these cancers are adenocarcinomas. Risk factors include increasing age, a diet high in red meats, obesity, inflammatory bowel disease, previous history of bowel cancer and genetic conditions such as familial adenomatous polyposis (FAP) and hereditary non-polyposis colorectal cancer (HNPCC). Common presenting complaints include a change in bowel habit, rectal bleeding and abdominal pain. Symptoms often vary in nature according to the site of the tumour: right-sided lesions usually present with iron deficiency anaemia (from chronic blood loss) and a palpable mass, while left-sided lesions present with pain, rectal bleeding and a change in bowel habit. Up to 40% of those with colorectal cancer first present with a complication of the tumour, e.g. obstruction. Diagnosis is made using a combination of lower GI endoscopy (with or without biopsy) and barium studies. The diagnosis may also be made when a laparotomy is carried out for acute obstruction. Treatment is largely dependent on the extent of disease and may be performed with either curative or palliative intent.

36. MANAGING BILIARY TRACT DISEASE (2)

A – Abdominal ultrasound

This patient has presented with the symptoms of biliary colic, a condition caused by obstruction of the gallbladder outlet or cystic duct by a gallstone. Gallstones are common in the Western population (affecting 50% of people over the age of 50), although many people remain asymptomatic. Women are more commonly affected than men, and there is an association with pregnancy and obesity. Stones are composed of cholesterol, bile pigment or both. Pain is usually felt in the right upper quadrant but may radiate to the back and scapulae. Symptoms are exacerbated by eating fatty foods, as this stimulates contraction of the gallbladder. Abdominal ultrasound is the investigation of choice for diagnosing gallstones. Only 10% of gallstones are radio-opaque (unlike 90% of renal stones). Complications of gallstones other than biliary colic include cholecystitis, cholangitis, empyema of the gallbladder, pancreatitis, gallstone ileus and gallbladder carcinoma. The treatment of biliary colic is symptomatic, with the patient referred for elective cholecystectomy.

37. PAEDIATRIC ORTHOPAEDICS (4)

D – Slipped upper femoral epiphysis

Slipped upper femoral epiphysis is a consequence of instability of the proximal femoral growth plate, resulting in the postero-lateral displacement of the femoral head in relation to the femur. It is a rare but important cause of hip pain in adolescents. Slipped upper femoral epiphysis commonly presents between the ages of 10 and 15, with boys and the left hip most commonly affected. The condition is bilateral in at least 20% of cases. Associations include hypothyroidism, Frohlich adiposogenital syndrome (characterized by obesity and hypogonadotrophic hypogonadism) and a tall stature. Slipped upper femoral epiphysis may present acutely after minimal trauma or have a more insidious presentation. Symptoms include hip, groin and knee pain, a limp, and an externally rotated and shortened leg. Acute cases may present with an inability to weight bear. The diagnosis may be made on X-ray (AP and lateral 'frog's leg' view), which may show widening of the growth plate and displacement of the femoral head. The management of slipped upper femoral epiphysis is bed rest (to prevent further slippage) and analgesia, until orthopaedic assessment is carried out. The management is then by surgical closure of the epiphysis (usually performed as a closed procedure with cannulated screws). The contralateral hip may be fixed at the same time. Complications include avascular necrosis of the femoral head (secondary to attempts at reduction), coxa vara (caused by fusion in the slipped position), chondrolysis (destruction of articular cartilage), premature epiphyseal fusion and secondary osteoarthritis.

Spontaneous haemarthrosis is an acute spontaneous bleed into a joint without a history of trauma. The knee is most commonly affected. Spontaneous haemarthrosis is most commonly seen with haemophilia. Recurrent haemarthroses result in damage to the joint and early osteoarthritis.

38. BACK PAIN (2)

E – Transfer patient to a specialist spinal centre

This patient has presented with cauda equina syndrome, a neurosurgical emergency in which there is an acute compression of multiple nerve roots below the level of the conus medullaris. Symptoms include acute bladder and bowel dysfunction, saddle and perineal anaesthesia, weakness of muscles innervated by the affected nerve roots, absent lower extremity reflexes and bilateral leg pain. Causes include central disc prolapse, trauma and metastatic disease. The diagnosis and cause can be confirmed on MRI (and less sensitively by CT and myelography); however, to prevent irreversible nerve damage, review by the specialist team must not be delayed in waiting for further investigation. Transfer of the patient to a specialist centre would be more appropriate. The mainstay of treatment is surgical decompression.

Cauda equina, from Latin *cauda* = tail + *equus* = horse.

39. UROLOGICAL CONDITIONS (1)

A – Atonic bladder

The atonic bladder in this case has resulted from autonomic neuropathy secondary to diabetes. Due to a lack of sensation of the desire to void, the bladder continues to enlarge until overflow incontinence occurs. This patient will need to be taught intermittent self-catheterization. Atonic bladder may occur after spinal injuries and lower motor neurone disease. Detrusor instability is the spontaneous contraction of the bladder during filling and results in urge incontinence. Benign prostatic hyperplasia can cause overflow incontinence secondary to bladder outflow obstruction but the patient will have the sensation of a full bladder or incomplete emptying. Urinary tract infections and bladder calculi are associated with irritative bladder symptoms such as frequency, urgency and dysuria.

40. GLASGOW COMA SCORE (2)

C – 3

The Glasgow coma scale is a widely used subjective scale used to assess and record a patient's conscious level. It is scored using three components: best eye response, best verbal response and best motor response (see the question, 'Glasgow coma score (1)').

In this case, the patient does not open his eyes at all (E1), makes no sound (V1) and makes no motor response (M1). Therefore his GCS is 3. Please note, the minimum GCS is 3, not 0, even when the patient is dead.

41. MANAGEMENT OF HERNIAS (1)

A – Conservative treatment unless symptoms change

This patient has presented with an incisional hernia. Incisional hernias are caused by a weakness in the abdominal wall at sites of previous abdominal incisions. They are a late complication in 10% of patients following abdominal surgery. Factors predisposing to an incisional hernia include poor surgical technique (too tight a closure), type of incision (vertical scars heal less well), post-operative wound infection, increasing age, obesity, chronic debilitating conditions such as diabetes, and steroid use. Incisional hernias are generally asymptomatic but may develop the same complications as other types of hernia, i.e. strangulation and obstruction. This patient is asymptomatic and therefore emergency surgery is not indicated. In view of her obesity and COPD, which would predispose to hernia recurrence, it would be safer to manage her conservatively unless circumstances change.

42. INVESTIGATING VASCULAR DISEASE (2)

E – Ultrasound Doppler

The symptom of calf pain on walking which is relieved by rest is suggestive of intermittent claudication; therefore imaging of the arterial system (largely peripheral) is required. Ultrasound Doppler is 90% sensitive for arterial disease and would be the first-line imaging investigation. Magnetic resonance angiogram is a fast, non-operator-dependent investigation, but has associated risks of contrast use. Digital subtraction angiography, although probably the most accurate investigation of the arterial system, carries with it the risks of contrast injection and would therefore be reserved for cases where intervention is deemed necessary.

43. MANAGING SKIN CONDITIONS (2)

C – Intravenous antibiotics

Erysipelas is a superficial streptococcal infection that is confined to a fascial compartment and is often found in the face or legs. It presents as a painful red swelling with a characteristically well-defined edge. Depending on the severity, erysipelas is treated with oral or intravenous antibiotics. Since the patient in this scenario is septic, intravenous antibiotics would be more appropriate. If erysipelas is not treated early, then infection can spread deeper and wider to become cellulitis or necrotizing fasciitis.

Erysipelas, from Greek *erusi* = red + *pelas* = skin.

44. MANAGING ABDOMINAL PAIN (4)

E – Laparotomy

This presentation is highly suggestive of a ruptured abdominal aortic aneurysm (AAA). The incidence of AAA is up to 5% in the over 60s and rupture accounts for around 2% of causes of death in men (AAA are less common in women and develop much later). The overall mortality associated with AAA is at least 60% (up to half die before they reach hospital) and is rising. The majority of AAAs are diagnosed incidentally. The classic presentation of a ruptured AAA is acute abdominal pain with hypotension and a pulsatile mass in the abdomen. The patient is often pale and sweaty, the mass may be tender, and an overlying bruit may be heard. Other presentations include back and flank pain (secondary to retroperitoneal haemorrhage – may be mistaken for renal colic) and circulatory collapse/cardiac arrest.

The investigation of a patient with a suspected AAA depends upon their stability. Insert two wide bore cannulae, take all routine bloods (including a cross match sample for 6 units) and start fluid resuscitation. Stable patients without evidence of haemodynamic instability are suitable for imaging, which may include abdominal X-ray (AAA is seen to be calcified in 75%), ultrasound examination (only useful if a diagnosis of AAA is not previously known) and CT (gives the most information). If the patient is unstable, an emergency operation is indicated, even if the patient is not adequately resuscitated. Operative mortality is 40% at 1 month. The main causes of post-operative death are renal and cardiac failure.

45. ACUTE LIMB ISCHAEMIA

E – Wet gangrene

This woman has presented with acute limb ischaemia, characterized by the six Ps: acute pain, pallor, paraesthesia, pulseless, paralysis, perishing coldness. This is a surgical emergency as irreversible damage can occur within 6 hours and there is loss of the limb in up to 40% of cases. Ischaemia can be caused by thrombus on pre-existing atherosclerotic areas (60%), emboli (30%), trauma, thrombosed aneurysm, dissecting aneurysm, prothrombotic states and intraarterial drug administration. Both an irregular cardiac rhythm and valvular dysfunction (congenital, rheumatic fever, post myocardial infarction) can lead to the formation of mural thrombus and subsequent emboli.

Wet gangrene occurs when there is infection within an area of dry gangrene, a feature of *chronic* ischaemia.

46. HAND DISORDERS (2)

E – Surgery

This patient has presented with a Dupuytren contracture, a flexion contracture of the hand caused by thickening of the connective tissue of the palmar aponeurosis. It most commonly affects the ring and little fingers, although sometimes there may be involvement of the other digits. The cause of Dupuytren's is largely unknown but it occurs in around 5% of the population. It typically presents after the age of 40 with men affected more than women. It has an association with manual labour, anti-epileptic medications (phenobarbitone, phenytoin), alcoholic liver disease, diabetes and hypothyroidism. Other areas of the body may also be affected such as the soles of the feet (Ledderhose disease) and the penis (Peyronie disease). In the early stages management is largely conservative but if function is affected then surgery is indicated. Surgery involves excising the thickened aponeurosis and would be followed by a period of splinting and physiotherapy to restore hand function. Re-thickening can occur so surgery may need to be repeated.

Guillaume Dupuytren, French anatomist and surgeon (1778–1835).
François Gigot de la Peyronie, French surgeon (1678–1747).
Georg Ledderhose, German surgeon (1855–1925).

47. THYROID DISEASE (4)

E – Primary myxoedema

The woman in this question presents with some classic features of an underactive thyroid. This, along with the lack of goitre, makes primary myxoedema the best answer. Primary myxoedema is also known as spontaneous atrophic hypothyroidism. It is characterized by an idiopathic reduction in the production of thyroid hormones. Features of hypothyroidism include a hoarse voice, constipation, feeling cold, weight gain, low mood, lethargy, coarse hair and dysmenorrhoea. The diagnosis of primary hypothyroidism is made by demonstrating a low T_4 (thyroxine) despite a high TSH (thyroid-stimulating hormone). Hypothyroidism is treated with daily thyroxine, which is taken for life.

Older patients with undiagnosed hypothyroidism, or those who do not take their medications, can present with features of severe hypothyroidism or a myxoedema coma. These include impaired consciousness, hypothermia, bradycardia and hypoglycaemia. Patients with a myxoedema coma should be transferred to intensive care for fluids, gentle re-warming and intravenous thyroid hormones. The mortality is 50%.

Haemorrhage into a thyroid cyst presents with acute neck pain and swelling. Haemorrhage can result in tracheal compression and stridor. If possible, aspiration of the cyst contents should be performed to alleviate tracheal compression and maintain airway patency. If aspiration is not possible, surgical intervention may be required.

Myxoedema, from Greek *myxa* = slime + *oedema* = swelling.

48. PAEDIATRIC SURGERY (4)

C – Nephroblastoma

A nephroblastoma, also known as Wilms tumour, is formed by the embryonic precursor to renal cells and can arise anywhere in the kidney. The incidence is 1 in 10,000 and it accounts for up to 20% of childhood malignancies. The typical age of presentation is 2–3 years, with boys being more commonly affected. Around 10% of cases of Wilms tumour are bilateral. It is associated with a deletion on the short arm of chromosome 11 and may be linked with other congenital anomalies such as aniridia (incomplete formation of the iris) and polycystic kidney disease. Presentation is usually vague (features include weight loss, anorexia and fever) and the abdominal mass is often found incidentally on examination. Diagnosis can be confirmed on ultrasound and CT. Nephrectomy and radiotherapy is the mainstay of treatment of localized disease, with chemotherapy in advanced disease. Nephroblastomas are pale grey with areas of haemorrhage on cross-section.

Neuroblastomas are tumours of the neural crest and most commonly occur in the adrenal medulla. The mass typically crosses the midline, unlike nephroblastomas which rarely do. Hepatoblastomas are rare primary liver cell cancers which present with a right-sided abdominal mass. Infantile polycystic kidney disease is a rare autosomal recessive condition that is bilateral. Lipomas are benign fatty tumours and are rarely symptomatic.

Max Wilms, German surgeon (1867–1918).

49. MANAGING COMMON FRACTURES (2)

C – 6 weeks

As a general rule, upper limb fractures in adults take 6–8 weeks to heal, while lower limb fractures take 12–16 weeks. These numbers are halved in children. Healing times are affected by fracture type and site, quality of local blood supply, amount of soft tissue interposition and amount of movement at the site of injury. Patient factors, such as anaemia, chronic illness and steroid use, will also have a bearing on healing.

50. STATISTICS (2)

D – 87.5%

The specificity is the ability of an investigation to detect a truly negative test result.

$$\text{Specificity} = \text{number of true negatives}/(\text{number of true negatives} + \text{number of false positives}) \times 100$$

In this case, 700 people who did not have tented T waves also did not have hyperkalaemia, i.e. of the 800 'negative' results, 700 were true negatives. Similarly, only 100 of the 200 people with 'tented T waves' truly had hyperkalaemia; in other words there were 100 true positives and 100 false positives.

Thus,

$$\text{Specificity} = 700/(700 + 100) \times 100 = 7/8 \times 100 = 87.5\%$$

For other useful formulas, see the question 'Statistics (1)'.

Practice Paper 5: Questions

1. PATHOLOGICAL FRACTURES

A 55-year-old woman presented to the emergency department with a fracture of the distal radius following a low-velocity injury. She was referred for a DEXA scan, which showed her bone density to be three standard deviations below the mean.

Which of the following has resulted in this patient's fracture?

A. Osteogenesis imperfecta
B. Osteomalacia
C. Osteopenia
D. Osteopetrosis
E. Osteoporosis

2. ABDOMINAL PAIN (13)

A 74-year-old man presents to the emergency department with a 6-hour history of colicky lower abdominal pain accompanied by gross abdominal distension. He has had similar episodes in the past that have been relieved by opening his bowels. Today he is not even able to pass flatus. Abdominal X-ray shows a grossly dilated loop of large bowel.

Which of the following is the most likely diagnosis?

A. Adhesions
B. Faecal impaction
C. Intussusception
D. Sigmoid volvulus
E. Strangulated inguinal hernia

3. AIRWAY MANAGEMENT (2)

You are called to see a 72-year-old man who has fallen on the ward two days post-laparotomy. On arrival, the patient appears to be unconscious and his breathing is noisy and laboured. His oxygen saturations are 76% on air.

Which of the following would be the next most appropriate step in your management?

A. Endotracheal intubation
B. Head-tilt chin-lift
C. Needle cricothyroidotomy
D. Supplemental oxygen
E. Surgical tracheostomy

4. MANAGEMENT OF HERNIAS (2)

A 56-year-old woman presents to the emergency department with an acutely painful lump in the right groin. She has vomited six times in the last hour and is also complaining of worsening abdominal pain. On examination, there is a grape-sized lump below and lateral to the pubic tubercle. It is warm, red and exquisitely tender. No cough impulse is felt.

What would be the best course of management?

A. Elective repair
B. Emergency repair
C. Observation alone
D. Prompt repair
E. Urgent repair

5. LOCAL ANAESTHETIC AGENTS (2)

A 56-year-old man is having a spinal anaesthetic for a lower limb operation as he has been told he is not fit enough for a general anaesthetic.

Which would be the most appropriate local anaesthetic agent?

A. Bupivacaine alone
B. Lidocaine
C. Lidocaine/prilocine mixture
D. Lidocaine with adrenaline
E. Prilocaine

6. COMPLICATIONS OF PANCREATITIS

A 65-year-old man is on the surgical ward being treated for pancreatitis. Initially he appeared to be improving, however on day 4 he develops fever and increasing epigastric pain. His serum C-reactive protein is noted to be rising.

Which of the following is the most likely cause?

A. Ascites
B. Gastrointestinal haemorrhage
C. Ileus
D. Infective pancreatic necrosis
E. Pancreatic pseudocyst

7. MANAGING ABDOMINAL TRAUMA

A 33-year-old man is brought into the emergency department following an assault with a baseball bat. He has bruising over the abdomen and right loin and complains of abdominal pain. On examination, his chest is clear with good air entry but his abdomen is rigid. On arrival, his heart rate is 140/min and blood pressure 90/60 mmHg. He is given O-negative blood in the resuscitation room but his observations remain unchanged.

What would be the next step in his management?

A. Diagnostic peritoneal lavage
B. Laparotomy
C. Urgent CT scan
D. Urgent intravenous urogram
E. Urgent ultrasound scan

8. CHEST PAIN

A 68-year-old man presents with acute lower chest and upper abdominal pain following an episode of vomiting. On examination, he has marked tenderness in the epigastrium and you note the presence of subcutaneous emphysema. ECG shows a sinus tachycardia with no ST segment changes, and a chest X-ray demonstrates mediastinal air.

Which of the following is the most likely diagnosis?

A. Boerhaave syndrome
B. Chest infection
C. Mallory-Weiss tear
D. Myocardial infarction
E. Pulmonary embolus

9. INTERPRETATION OF LIVER FUNCTION TESTS

A 34-year-old woman is being investigated for jaundice. Investigations show elevations of bilirubin, aspartate transaminase and alkaline phosphatase in the blood. Gamma GT levels are normal. There is no urobilinogen in the urine.

Which of the following conditions would be compatible with the above results?

A. Gallstones
B. Gilbert syndrome
C. Hereditary spherocytosis
D. Liver metastasis
E. Viral hepatitis

10. DIARRHOEA

A 37-year-old woman presents to the GP with a 3-week history of frequent, loose motions. She is very tired and complains of muscle weakness.

A subsequent colonoscopy demonstrates a 1.5 cm sessile growth that has multiple projections. The remainder of the colon was unremarkable.

What is the most likely diagnosis?

A. Adenomatous polyp
B. Colorectal carcinoma
C. Infective colitis
D. Pseudomembranous colitis
E. Villous adenoma

11. ABDOMINAL PAIN (14)

A 45-year-old man presents with episodic upper abdominal pain, severe heartburn, episodes of dark vomitus and diarrhoea. He has been taking over-the-counter indigestion medication with no relief. On endoscopy, he has multiple ulcers throughout the duodenum, some of which are large.

Which of the following is most likely to have caused this?

A. Alcohol
B. Aspirin use
C. Gastrinoma
D. *Helicobacter pylori* infection
E. Smoking

12. ANATOMY OF HERNIAS (3)

Which term best fits the description of hernia given below?

A hernia that contains a 'W' loop of intestine within its sac.

A. Gluteal
B. Inguinal
C. Maydl
D. Obturator
E. Sciatic

13. RENAL STONES

A 65-year-old man presents to the emergency department with a 3-hour history of left loin pain radiating to the left groin. He is known to have benign prostatic hypertrophy and recurrent urinary tract infections. The intravenous urogram (IVU) shows a standing column on the left.

Which of the following types of stone is most likely to have caused his symptoms?

A. Calcium
B. Cholesterol
C. Cysteine
D. Magnesium ammonium phosphate
E. Uric acid

14. HYPERSENSITIVITY

A 34-year-old man is receiving a blood transfusion after a large upper gastrointestinal bleed. Soon after his transfusion starts he develops a high fever and chest pains. He is found to have a heart rate of 120/min and a blood pressure of 102/68 mmHg.

Which type of hypersensitivity reaction is this?

A. Type I hypersensitivity
B. Type II hypersensitivity
C. Type III hypersensitivity
D. Type IV hypersensitivity
E. Type V hypersensitivity

15. CLASSIFICATION OF HERNIAS (2)

A 39-year-old man presents to the emergency department with a painful lump in the groin. He tells you that this lump has been present on and off for a few months and has previously been asymptomatic. Today, the lump has become painful. On examination, there is an erythematous, tender, irreducible lump above and medial to the pubic tubercle. The patient denies abdominal pain, vomiting or constipation.

Which is the best descriptive term for the hernia above?

A. Incarcerated hernia
B. Perforated hernia
C. Richter hernia
D. Sliding hernia
E. Strangulated hernia

16. EPONYMOUS FRACTURES (2)

A 65-year-old woman presents to the emergency department with right wrist pain following a fall onto an outstretched hand. An X-ray shows a fracture of the distal radius with volar displacement of the distal fragment. There is no intra-articular involvement.

Which of the following would be the most appropriate term to describe this fracture?

A. Barton fracture
B. Colles fracture
C. Galeazzi fracture
D. Monteggia fracture
E. Smith fracture

17. X-RAY CHANGES IN OSTEOARTHRITIS

A 45-year-old woman attends the orthopaedic follow-up clinic to receive the results of a knee X-ray. She has been getting increasing pain in the left knee, aggravated by walking.

Which of the following changes on X-ray would most suggest a diagnosis of osteoarthritis?

A. Joint subluxation
B. Juxta-articular erosions
C. Narrowed joint space
D. Soft tissue swelling
E. Subchondral sclerosis

18. PAEDIATRIC ORTHOPAEDICS (5)

A 4-year-old boy is brought into hospital by his mother. He has been having episodes of intermittent high fever associated with a generalized non-itchy, pink rash over the body and swelling of the knees on and off for the last 2 weeks.

What is the most likely diagnosis?

A. Juvenile pauciarticular arthritis
B. Juvenile polyarticular arthritis
C. Septic arthritis
D. Still's disease
E. Transient synovitis

19. INVESTIGATING BREAST DISEASE (2)

A 22-year old woman presents to the GP complaining of a 2-week history of milky discharge from both her breasts. She is otherwise well. Clinical examination of the breasts is unremarkable and a pregnancy test is negative.

Which of the following investigations would be indicated in the first instance?

A. Dopamine levels
B. Fine needle aspiration
C. Mammogram
D. MRI of the breast
E. Prolactin levels

20. COMPLICATIONS OF THYROIDECTOMY

You are called to see a 52-year-old woman who has just undergone a thyroidectomy. She complains of a 20-minute history of neck pain and shortness of breath. A rapidly expanding mass is noted around the operation site.

Which of the following would you do next?

A. Anaesthetic review
B. Bedside opening of incision
C. Book next available theatre slot
D. Intravenous antibiotics
E. Laryngoscopy

21. ANORECTAL DISEASE (4)

A 49-year-old woman presents with a 4-month history of perianal itching with occasional mucous discharge. She is otherwise well. On examination, large fleshy pink lesions are seen around the anus.

What is the most likely diagnosis?

A. Condylomata lata
B. Condylomata acuminata
C. Anal carcinoma
D. Rectal prolapse
E. Haemorrhoids

22. SKIN LESIONS (5)

A 56-year-old man presents to the GP with a lesion on the tip of his right middle finger which has developed over the past week since he pricked his finger on a thorn in the garden. On examination, the lesion is 1 cm in size, dark red in colour and bleeds easily.

What is the most likely diagnosis?

A. Cavernous haemangioma
B. Ganglion
C. Granuloma annulare
D. Kaposi sarcoma
E. Pyogenic granuloma

23. KNEE CONDITIONS (3)

A 14-year-old girl presents to the GP surgery complaining of right knee pain which occurs after gymnastics training. She is otherwise well. On examination, there is a full range of movement at the right knee joint and a small tender lump over the upper tibia.

What is the most likely diagnosis?

A. Baker cyst
B. Bipartite patella
C. Chondromalacia patellae
D. Dislocation of the patella
E. Osgood–Schlatter disease

24. GROIN LUMPS (5)

A 20-year-old man presents to the GP with a 2-day history of severe pain and swelling in his right testicle. On examination, there is a purulent discharge present at the urethral meatus and the right testicle is tender to palpation.

What is the most likely diagnosis?

A. Epididymo-orchitis
B. Mumps orchitis

C. Testicular cancer

D. Testicular torsion

E. Varicocele

25. JAUNDICE (5)

A 65-year-old man has been brought into hospital by his wife. She is concerned as he has become increasingly yellow in colour and has unintentional weight loss. The patient denies any pain. On examination he is jaundiced and has a palpable mass in the right upper quadrant.

What is the most likely diagnosis?

A. Cholangiocarcinoma

B. Gallstones

C. Gastric carcinoma

D. Hepatocellular carcinoma

E. Pancreatic carcinoma

26. URETHRAL INJURY

A 21-year-old man is brought into the emergency department with penile pain and swelling following a fall onto the crossbar of a bicycle. On examination, the penis is oedematous and bruised and there is blood at the urethral meatus. He is otherwise stable.

Which of the following investigations is indicated?

A. Bladder scan and urethral catheterization

B. CT abdomen and pelvis

C. Cystoscopy

D. Intravenous urogram

E. Retrograde urethrogram

27. NECK LUMPS (5)

A 6-year-old girl is brought to the GP by her father with a smooth lump in the midline of her neck. She is otherwise well. On examination, there is a 1 cm painless, fluctuant swelling which moves upwards on swallowing and on tongue protrusion.

What is the most likely diagnosis?

A. Branchial cyst

B. Chemodectoma

C. Cystic hygroma

D. Thyroid adenoma

E. Thyroglossal cyst

28. EAR DISEASE (2)

A 44-year-old man presents to the GP practice complaining of a 2-month history of painless, purulent, foul-smelling discharge from his right ear.

His hearing is gradually getting worse. On examination, there is no obvious abnormality externally.

Which of the following is the most likely cause of his symptoms?

A. Acute otitis media
B. Cerumen
C. Cholesteatoma
D. Glue ear
E. Swimmer's ear

29. TRAUMA

A 33-year-old man who was travelling on his motorbike has been hit by a car at 50 miles per hour. He is brought into the emergency department by his friend and it is noted that his left leg appears deformed. His pulse is 120/min and his blood pressure 100/65 mmHg.

What is the next step in your management?

A. Assess the patient's breathing
B. Give blood
C. Give fluids
D. Immobilize the patient
E. Splint the left leg

30. ABDOMINAL PAIN (15)

A 27-year-old man presents to the emergency department with severe epigastric pain which started soon after eating his lunch. On examination, the upper abdomen is rigid. The patient says he has recently been suffering from indigestion which started after medical treatment for a meniscal injury to his knee.

Which of the following medications could have contributed to his condition?

A. Aspirin
B. Codeine
C. Gaviscon
D. Omeprazole
E. Paracetamol

31. CUTANEOUS MALIGNANCIES (3)

A 62-year-old man presents to the GP with a lesion on his left forehead that has been present for 6 months. It has recently begun to ulcerate. On examination, there is a 1 cm raised, hyperkeratotic, crusty lesion with raised edges.

What is the most likely diagnosis?

A. Actinic keratosis
B. Basal cell carcinoma

C. Bowen disease

D. Keratoacanthoma

E. Squamous cell carcinoma

32. MANAGING ENDOCRINE DISEASE (2)

A 37-year-old woman presents to the emergency department following a faint after standing up from a sitting position. She did not lose consciousness during this episode but reported feeling 'dizzy and lightheaded'. She has no significant past medical history. On examination you notice multiple areas of skin depigmentation but increased pigmentation in the palmar creases and on the elbows.

Which of the following is the best management for her condition?

A. Desmopressin

B. Hydrocortisone and fludrocortisone

C. Octreotide

D. Spironolactone

E. Thyroidectomy

33. PAEDIATRIC SURGERY (5)

A 7-day-old preterm boy develops vomiting and bloody diarrhoea. On examination, his abdomen is grossly distended and discoloured. His temperature is 39.5°C.

What is the most likely diagnosis?

A. Exomphalos

B. Gastroenteritis

C. Gastroschisis

D. Meconium ileus

E. Necrotizing enterocolitis

34. UROLOGICAL CONDITIONS (2)

A 4-year-old girl is referred to the urology clinic by the GP as she has been having recurrent urinary tract infections. Examination of the child is unremarkable.

Which of the following is most likely to be causing the problem?

A. Hydronephrosis

B. Pelvic kidney

C. Posterior urethral valve

D. Renal agenesis

E. Vesica-ureteric reflux

35. FEMORAL NECK FRACTURES (2)

An 81-year-old woman from a nursing home is brought into the emergency department following a fall. She is complaining of pain in her left hip. On examination, her left leg is shortened and externally rotated. The home tells you this woman has dementia but is able to mobilize independently with a frame. An X-ray shows a displaced intracapsular femoral neck fracture.

Which of the following would be the most suitable management option?

A. Allow the patient to try to mobilize
B. Dynamic hip screw
C. Hemiarthroplasty
D. Open reduction and internal fixation
E. Total hip replacement

36. MANAGING BILIARY TRACT DISEASE (3)

A 45-year-old woman presents to the emergency department with a 12-hour history of worsening right upper abdominal pain and vomiting. On examination, she is locally peritonitic in the right upper quadrant. Her temperature is 38.1°C.

Which of the following treatment options would be indicated in the first instance?

A. Cholecystectomy
B. Intravenous antibiotics
C. Intravenous steroids
D. Intravenous proton pump inhibitor
E. Percutaneous drainage of the gallbladder

37. MANAGING UROLOGICAL DISEASE (3)

A 59-year-old man presents with an 8-month history of urinary hesitancy, poor stream and the sensation of incomplete bladder emptying. He is otherwise well. On examination, his prostate is homogeneously enlarged and smooth.

Which of the following interventions would be indicated?

A. Bladder neck incision
B. Brachytherapy
C. External beam radiotherapy
D. Radical prostatectomy
E. Transurethral resection of prostate

38. STATISTICS (3)

A new blood test has been produced to help diagnose suspected tumours of the membranous urethra. Of a study sample of 100 patients, 20 are known to have cancer of the membranous urethra. The blood test suggested that 30 people had the tumour, but of these only 15 were true positives.

What is the positive predictive value of this test?

A. 25%
B. 50%
C. 75%
D. 90%
E. 100%

39. MANAGEMENT OF VENOUS DISEASE (2)

A 45-year-old male coach driver presents to the emergency department with a 3-day history of a swollen left leg and some shortness of breath. On examination, the left calf is swollen and tender. The pedal pulses are palpable and the foot is warm.

What would be the most appropriate initial management?

A. Elevation, rest and NSAIDs
B. Emergency surgery
C. Intravenous heparin
D. Subcutaneous low molecular weight heparin
E. Warfarin

40. MANAGEMENT OF AORTIC ANEURYSMS

A 72-year-old man who has no past medical history of note has been referred to you by his GP. His GP found an incidental non-tender expansile mass in his abdomen. An ultrasound scan demonstrates an abdominal aortic aneurysm that is 5 cm in diameter.

What is the best course of management?

A. Admit for emergency repair
B. Commence on antihypertensives and advise to see GP if he develops abdominal pain
C. Organize an elective repair
D. Repeat an ultrasound scan in 3 months
E. Repeat an ultrasound scan in 1 year

41. MANAGING SKIN CONDITIONS (3)

A 34-year-old man is brought to the emergency department. Three days ago he suffered an insect bite to the upper leg; he is now complaining of severe pain in the thigh, fever and vomiting. On examination of the thigh, there is marked, spreading erythema with areas of blistering and skin necrosis.

Which of the following is the best course of management?

A. Intravenous antibiotics alone
B. Intravenous antibiotics and surgical debridement
C. Intravenous steroids
D. Oral antibiotics
E. Skin biopsy

42. COLORECTAL OPERATIONS (2)

A 56-year-old man presents to the emergency department with a 3-hour history of severe abdominal pain and vomiting. On examination, the abdomen is rigid. A CT scan confirms free air in the peritoneum and a perforation of a sigmoid diverticulum.

What is the most appropriate operation?

A. Abdominoperineal resection
B. Extended right hemicolectomy
C. Hartmann procedure
D. Left hemicolectomy
E. Right hemicolectomy

43. TUMOUR STAGING

A 59-year-old woman has recently had a resection of a sigmoid adenocarcinoma. The pathology report said that the tumour invaded through the bowel wall but there was no evidence of lymph node involvement.

Which of the following best describes this stage of tumour?

A. Dukes A
B. Dukes B
C. Dukes C1
D. Dukes C2
E. Dukes D

44. HAND DISORDERS (3)

A 37-year-old woman presents with a 2-day history of increasing pain and swelling of the right middle finger. She tells you she sustained a minor cut to the inner surface of the finger 4 days ago. On examination, the finger is grossly swollen, red and held in the flexed position.

Which of the following is the most likely diagnosis?

A. Fascial space infection
B. Felon
C. Infective tenosynovitis
D. Paronychia
E. Whitlow

45. GASTROINTESTINAL POLYPS (2)

A 27-year-old man presents to the emergency department following an episode of vomiting blood. On examination he is haemodynamically stable and is noted to have multiple freckles around his lips and mouth. A subsequent endoscopy demonstrates multiple polyps throughout the duodenum which are confirmed as benign.

What is the most likely morphology of the polyps?

A. Adenomatous polyp
B. Hamartomatous polyp
C. Juvenile polyp
D. Metaplastic polyp
E. Pseudo-polyp

46. BACK PAIN (3)

A 64-year-old man presents to the GP practice with a 2-month history of intermittent episodes of lower back pain radiating to both legs on walking. His symptoms are relieved by sitting or leaning forward. He has no back pain at rest. Examination is unremarkable.

Which of the following is the most likely cause of his symptoms?

A. Intermittent claudication
B. Lumbar spondylosis
C. Lumbar spondylolisthesis
D. Spinal stenosis
E. Spinal tumour

47. URINARY TRACT INFECTION

A 24-year-old woman with no past medical history of note comes to see you at the GP practice complaining of a 2-day history of urinary frequency together with a stinging sensation on passing urine. She is systemically well.

Which of the following organisms is most likely to have caused her symptoms?

A. *Candida albicans*
B. *Escherichia coli*
C. Herpes simplex
D. *Proteus mirabilis*
E. *Pseudomonas aeruginosa*

48. MANAGING COMMON FRACTURES (3)

A 27-year-old man was admitted to the ward after sustaining a right tibia and fibula fracture in a road traffic accident. He is currently in an above-knee backslab with the leg resting on a pillow, awaiting consultant review in the morning. You are called to the ward by the nurse saying the patient is in severe pain despite having morphine 2 hours ago. When you arrive at the ward the patient is crying in pain and complaining of an inability to move his toes.

Which of the following is the most appropriate measure to take?

A. Administer further analgesia and call senior orthopaedic doctor on call
B. Complete the cast to give more stability to the fracture

C. Elevate the limb further

D. Prescribe more regular analgesia and review in the morning

E. Remove backslab as a temporary measure and review in the morning

49. UPPER LIMB NERVE LESIONS (4)

A 17-year-old boy presents with severe left shoulder pain following a tackle during a rugby match. On examination, the contour of the left shoulder is flattened and the humeral head is palpable just under the clavicle. There is also sensory loss at the upper lateral aspect of the arm.

Which nerve has most likely been affected?

A. Accessory nerve

B. Axillary nerve

C. Long thoracic nerve

D. Median nerve

E. Radial nerve

50. ULCERS (4)

A 27-year-old man is admitted to the high dependency ward having sustained a significant head injury. Two days later he starts vomiting blood.

Which of the following is the most likely cause?

A. Curling ulcer

B. Cushing ulcer

C. Decubitus ulcer

D. Dendritic ulcer

E. Martorell's ulcer

Practice Paper 5: Answers

1. PATHOLOGICAL FRACTURES

E – Osteoporosis

Osteoporosis is a reduction in bone density, which can result in low-velocity fractures, commonly of the distal radius, vertebrae and pelvis. It is diagnosed on DEXA (dual energy X-ray absorptiometry) scan by demonstrating a density that is 2.5 standard deviations below the mean. Osteopenia also describes a reduction in bone density but is not as severe as osteoporosis. On DEXA scanning, density will be between 1 and 2.5 standard deviations below the mean. In osteomalacia there is reduction in skeletal mass secondary to abnormal mineralization of the bone, which can be diagnosed biochemically and on bone biopsy. In osteopetrosis there is overgrowth and sclerosis of bone which can grow into the medullary canal. This bone is brittle and susceptible to fractures. Osteogenesis imperfecta is a genetic bone disorder resulting from collagen deficiency; there is subsequent bone fragility. It is usually inherited in an autosomal dominant manner and presents in infancy with frequent fractures.

2. ABDOMINAL PAIN (13)

D – Sigmoid volvulus

A volvulus is the twisting of a bowel loop around its mesenteric axis. Sigmoid volvulus is a well-documented cause of large bowel obstruction, accounting for up to 10% of cases. It is associated with chronic constipation and the development of an elongated, atonic segment of bowel (megacolon) which may easily twist around the mesenteric axis. The risk of this is that it forms a 'closed loop' obstruction which can result in infarction, perforation and peritonitis. Volvulus is more common at the extremes of age and is most common in elderly men. Presentation is with symptoms and signs of bowel obstruction which may have an acute or insidious onset. The diagnosis can usually be made on abdominal X-ray, which shows a twisted, dilated loop of bowel (the 'coffee bean' sign). The mainstay of treatment is decompression of the volvulus. In most cases this can be performed using a flatus tube which is inserted into the colon via the rectum. Sometimes decompression may be achieved by means of a barium enema. If conservative management fails, or there are signs of bowel ischaemia or perforation, then surgery is required.

Sigmoid volvulus is recurrent in around 50% of those treated conservatively. Volvulus may also occur in the caecum (25% of cases) and most commonly affects the terminal ileum and ascending colon. It is associated with a congenital abnormality where there is an incomplete rotation of the midgut causing a failure in the attachment of the caecum to the posterior abdominal wall. The majority of cases are treated surgically. Small bowel volvulus is rare in the UK and is associated with tumours and adhesions. The condition is most common in Africa and associated with a high roughage diet and the loading of the small bowel with vegetable matter. Volvuli of the stomach do occur, but are very rare.

Volvulus, from Latin *volvere* = to roll.

3. AIRWAY MANAGEMENT (2)

B – Head-tilt chin-lift

This patient has noisy breathing, suggestive of his inability to maintain his own airway. The easiest and quickest way to open the airway is by performing a head-tilt chin-lift manoeuvre: one hand is placed on the forehead to tilt the head backwards; the other hand is placed under the chin and lifted to help keep the mouth open. This posture is known as the 'sniffing the morning air' position. Another airway-opening manoeuvre, which can be used if the patient is unconscious, is the jaw thrust. This is done by placing two fingers under the angle of the mandible on both sides, with the thumbs on the patient's chin, and lifting the jaw upwards. Supplemental oxygen may then be given. If the patient is still unable to maintain the airway in this manner, then endotracheal intubation by an experienced person may need to be considered.

Endotracheal intubation is the placement of a tube in the trachea in order to secure and provide a definitive airway. Indications include airway obstruction not responding to simple interventions, respiratory failure and respiratory arrest. In the trauma setting, endotracheal intubation may be used in cases of smoke inhalation injuries where oedema of the upper airways is expected, and in those with severe pulmonary contusions. A needle cricothyroidotomy is an emergency procedure, performed by passing a wide-bore cannula through the skin and cricothyroid membrane, just below the thyroid cartilage (Adam's apple). It is used only in cases where oral and nasal intubation is not possible, e.g. in facial trauma or repeated failed attempts at endotracheal intubation. The needle cricothyroidotomy is a temporary measure and will allow for around 30 minutes of ventilation, giving time for a more permanent airway to be created. A surgical tracheostomy is the formation of a definitive airway, via the trachea, used when endotracheal intubation is not possible. It may be performed as an open or percutaneous procedure.

4. MANAGEMENT OF HERNIAS (2)

B – Emergency repair
In order of increasing priority, the options for managing hernias are observation, elective repair, prompt repair, urgent repair and emergency repair. Elective repairs are done at a mutually convenient time and prompt surgery is done within specific time limits. Urgent operations are done as soon as possible within 24 hours following adequate resuscitation. Emergency procedures are performed immediately for life-saving procedures where resuscitation is carried out at the same time as surgery.

This woman presents with a femoral hernia with features of obstruction. This requires emergency repair. Femoral hernias without features of strangulation or obstruction should still be repaired urgently, as there is a 50% risk of strangulation within a month.

5. LOCAL ANAESTHETIC AGENTS (2)

A – Bupivacaine alone
Bupivacaine is a longer-acting anaesthetic that can be used without adrenaline for spinal or epidural anaesthesia. Bupivacaine can also be injected into surgical wounds with adrenaline to reduce post-operative pain for up to 20 hours. The maximum dose of bupivacaine is 2 mg/kg. A mixture of bupivacaine and lidocaine is used for carpal tunnel surgery as it allows rapid onset of anaesthesia and longer-acting post-operative analgesia. Bupivacaine is contraindicated for intravenous regional anaesthesia (such as Bier block) as it is cardiotoxic.

Before manipulation of a Colles fracture, regional anaesthesia of the upper limb is required. This technique is known as a Bier block. A Bier block is performed by first squeezing the blood out of the limb, then inflating a tourniquet around the upper arm and injecting intravenous prilocaine into the arm distal to the tourniquet. The tourniquet prevents local anaesthetic from leaving the arm and blood from entering. Prilocaine is the best local anaesthetic to use for this procedure as it is the least cardiotoxic.

For uses of lidocaine see the question 'Local anaesthetic agents (1)'.
August Bier, German surgeon (1861–1949).

6. COMPLICATIONS OF PANCREATITIS

D – Infective pancreatic necrosis
Following inflammation of the pancreas, necrosis can develop. The diagnosis of pancreatic necrosis is suggested by an increasing C-reactive protein and worsening pain; this is confirmed on CT scanning with or without fine needle aspiration. Up to 70% of cases become infected. The treatment of pancreatic necrosis is surgical debridement and drainage. A *pancreatic pseudocyst* is a parapancreatic collection of pancreatic juices

and develops around 4 weeks after acute pancreatitis. This can rupture into the peritoneal cavity causing ascites. Ileus and haemorrhage are also complications of pancreatitis, together with abscess formation. Systemic complications include acute respiratory distress syndrome, pulmonary oedema, renal dysfunction, shock, disseminated intravascular coagulation and hypocalcaemia.

7. MANAGING ABDOMINAL TRAUMA

B – Laparotomy

This patient has suffered blunt abdominal trauma and is haemodynamically unstable despite blood resuscitation. This is an indication for an urgent laparotomy, to identify and manage the site of bleeding. From the history there are no obvious sites of blood loss, so it can only be assumed that it is being lost into the abdomen. Had the patient been haemodynamically stable and not requiring blood, there would be time for further investigations to identify the source of bleeding. Both ultrasound and CT are useful to determine organ damage and identify fluid in the abdomen. An intravenous urogram can be used in stable patients to determine injury of the renal tract specifically. Diagnostic peritoneal lavage is used in the multiply injured patient where there is uncertainty about the presence of abdominal injury. It is largely being replaced by bedside ultrasound scanning (FAST scanning).

FAST scan = Focussed Assessment with Sonography for Trauma.

8. CHEST PAIN

A – Boerhaave syndrome

Boerhaave syndrome describes spontaneous transmural rupture of the oesophagus, often associated with forceful vomiting. The most common site of rupture is the left posterolateral wall of the lower third of the oesophagus. Boerhaave syndrome is characterized by Mackler's triad: vomiting, lower thoracic pain and subcutaneous emphysema. Common presenting features include acute abdominal and chest pain, shortness of breath, and difficulty swallowing and coughing. There is usually a history of forceful vomiting or excessive consumption of food or alcohol. Boerhaave syndrome is most common in middle-aged men. An erect chest X-ray will be abnormal in 90%, the most common sign being a pleural effusion. The diagnosis is confirmed with a Gastrografin swallow. Treatment includes intravenous fluids, antibiotics and prompt surgical repair (although cervical oesophageal perforations may be managed conservatively). Complications of Boerhaave syndrome include septicaemia, mediastinitis and pneumomediastinum. There is an overall mortality rate of around 35%. The prognosis is best if treatment is carried out within the first 12 hours of rupture and worsens with increasing time intervals thereafter. The majority of cases of oesophageal rupture are iatrogenic and caused while performing an oesophagogastroduodenoscopy (OGD), although the overall risk of perforation at OGD is low (<1%). A Mallory–Weiss tear is a superficial laceration in the lower oesophagus that results in bleeding.

Herman Boerhaave, Dutch physician (1668–1738).

9. INTERPRETATION OF LIVER FUNCTION TESTS

A – Gallstones

Jaundice (also known as *icterus*) describes the yellow discolouration of the skin and mucous membranes secondary to increased serum bilirubin levels. It is usually clinically apparent when levels reach 40 μmol/L.

Jaundice may be classified as: (i) pre-hepatic (e.g. hereditary spherocytosis and Gilbert syndrome) where there is an inability of the liver to handle an excess amount of bilirubin being produced; (ii) hepatic (e.g. viral hepatitis and liver metastasis) caused by a primary failure of the hepatocytes to metabolise or excrete bilirubin; and (iii) post-hepatic (e.g. gallstones and carcinoma of the head of the pancreas) caused by the obstruction of bile ducts.

The following table summarizes the abnormalities found in each type of jaundice.

	Pre-hepatic	Hepatic	Post-hepatic
Serum bilirubin	High	High	High
Urine bilirubin	Absent	Normal/high	High
Conjugated bilirubin	Normal	Normal/low	High
Unconjugated bilirubin	Normal/high	Normal/reduced	Normal
Urobilinogen	Normal/high	Normal/reduced	Low
AST/ALT	Normal	Very high	Normal/high
ALP	Normal	Normal/high	Very high
Gamma GT	Normal	Very high	Normal/high
Urine colour	Normal	Normal/dark	Dark
Stool colour	Normal	Normal	Pale

10. DIARRHOEA

E – Villous adenoma

Villous adenomas are large polyps which look like sea anemones. Villous adenomas secrete mucus and potassium, hence they can present with diarrhoea and features of hypokalaemia (muscle weakness, myalgia and arrhythmias). Of all the rectal polyps, the villous adenoma has the highest potential for malignant change, so it must be removed.

Adenomatous polyps are benign polyps that have the potential to undergo malignant change. Because of this potential it is important that such polyps are removed. Multiple adenomatous polyps are found in familial adenomatous polyposis, a condition that predisposes to colorectal cancer.

Villous, from Latin *villus* = tuft of hair.

11. ABDOMINAL PAIN (14)

C – Gastrinoma

Peptic ulcers result from an imbalance between gastric acid secretion and mucosal barrier protection. All of the conditions listed are risk factors for the development of peptic ulceration; however, the presence of multiple ulceration in multiple sites, large ulcers and concomitant diarrhoea should alert the clinician to the presence of an underlying gastrinoma. A gastrinoma is a gastrin-producing tumour which results in an increase in the basal production of gastric acid with subsequent peptic ulceration. Ulceration may be severe, recurrent and refractory to treatment. Gastrinomas most commonly occur in the pancreas and duodenum, and more than 50% are malignant. The triad of a gastrin-producing tumour, gastric hypersecretion and severe peptic ulceration is known as the Zollinger-Ellison syndrome. This syndrome is the cause of around 0.1% of peptic ulceration. Treatment includes the use of proton pump inhibitors and resection of the tumour. Pancreatic gastrinomas may be the result of MEN I syndrome, a multiple endocrine neoplasia which affects the parathyroid gland, anterior pituitary gland and pancreatic islet cells.

Robert Milton Zollinger, American surgeon (1903–1992).

Edwin Homer Ellison, American surgeon (1918–1970).

12. ANATOMY OF HERNIAS (3)

C – Maydl hernia

A Maydl hernia is one that contains a 'W' loop of intestine, where the middle segment is liable to become strangulated.

Other hernias include:

Amyand hernia	→	contains the appendix within its sac
Gluteal hernia	→	protrudes through the greater sciatic foramen
Littre hernia	→	contains a Meckel diverticulum
Obturator hernia	→	protrudes through the obturator canal
Sciatic hernia	→	protrudes through the lesser sciatic foramen
Spigelian hernia	→	protrudes through the semilunar line

Obturator hernias pass through the obturator canal in the upper thigh, especially in older women. These hernias typically incarcerate and interfere with the obturator nerve, which supplies sensation to the medial thigh.

A Spigelian hernia – or spontaneous lateral ventral hernia – describes herniation through the semilunar line, which is a curved tendinous insertion that corresponds to the lateral border of the rectus abdominus muscle and is formed by the aponeuroses of the internal oblique, external oblique and transversus muscles. Spigelian hernias tend to occur below the level of the umbilicus. They are small and develop in the over 50s. They can present with diffuse pain around the area. There is a high risk of strangulation so these hernias should be repaired.

Claudius Amyand, English surgeon (1680–1740).
Alexis Littre, French anatomist (1685–1726).
Karel Maydl, Austrian surgeon (1853–1903).
Adriaan van den Spiegel, Flemish anatomist (1578–1625).

13. RENAL STONES

D – Magnesium ammonium phosphate

Magnesium ammonium phosphate stones, also known as struvite stones, are associated with chronic urinary tract infections (UTIs) caused by Gram-negative rods which can split urea into ammonium (*Pseudomonas, Proteus*). They account for 15% of renal calculi. Benign prostatic hypertrophy is a risk factor for the development of recurrent chronic UTIs as it can result in incomplete bladder emptying and stasis of urine. Calcium stones are the most common type of renal calculus (75%) and are associated with hyperparathyroidism, diuretic use and increased gut absorption of calcium (often familial). Uric acid stones are associated with gout and malignancy. Cysteine calculi are rare. Cholesterol is the main component of most gallstones.

14. HYPERSENSITIVITY

B – Type II hypersensitivity

Hypersensitivity reactions are classified using the Gell and Coombs system as follows:

Type I (anaphylactic)	→	IgE-mediated from allergen exposure
Type II (cytotoxic)	→	antibody-mediated
Type III (complexes)	→	immune complex-mediated
Type IV (delayed)	→	sensitised T-cell mediated
Type V (stimulatory)	→	stimulatory anti-receptor antibody mediated

This man is having an acute haemolytic reaction due to ABO incompatibility, which is an example of a type II hypersensitivity reaction. In type II hypersensitivity reactions, autoantibodies bind to the cell surfaces. This results in autoantibody-mediated destruction of cells. Other examples of type II hypersensitivity reactions include haemolytic disease of the newborn and autoimmune thrombocytopenia.

Type I hypersensitivity (anaphylactic) reactions occur when exposure to certain allergens results in IgE-mediated secretion of inflammatory mediators by basophils and mast cells. These inflammatory mediators, such as histamine and prostaglandins, result in vasodilatation and smooth muscle contraction, and symptoms range from mild irritation to anaphylactic shock and death. Treatment is with adrenaline, antihistamines (chlorphenamine) and steroids. Examples of type I hypersensitivity reactions include allergic asthma, hay fever (allergic rhinitis), and peanut allergies.

Type III hypersensitivity reactions are mediated by immune complexes (antigen-antibody complexes). Immune complexes can deposit in various sites in the body and result in localized tissue damage via complement activation. Examples of immune complex damage include glomerulonephritis following a streptococcal throat infection, rheumatic fever and systemic lupus erythematosus.

Type IV hypersensitivity reactions are known as delayed type reactions as features can take days to develop. T cells can become sensitised by certain allergens and this results in cytotoxic T cell-mediated cell damage. Examples of type IV hypersensitivity reactions include contact dermatitis (e.g. to nickel) and transplant rejection.

Type V (stimulatory) hypersensitivity reactions describe the presence of antibodies that bind to cell receptors and either stimulate or prevent stimulation of the receptor. Examples include Graves disease (a stimulatory response of autoantibodies binding to the TSH receptor of the thyroid gland) and myasthenia gravis (an inhibitory response from autoantibodies that bind to acetylcholine receptors at the neuromuscular junction).

Robin Coombs, British immunologist (1921–2006).
Philip Gell, British immunologist (1914–2001).

15. CLASSIFICATION OF HERNIAS (2)

C – Richter hernia

This man has a direct inguinal hernia that shows features of a Richter hernia. A Richter hernia describes strangulation of one sidewall of the bowel within a hernia sac. (By comparison, a strangulated hernia describes strangulation of the entire lumen of the bowel.) Richter hernias result in the features of strangulation (a painful, erythematous lump) but without the characteristics of obstruction.

A hernia is incarcerated when adhesions develop between the hernia sac and its contents, resulting in a painless irreducible lump which has no cough impulse. Incarcerated hernias predispose to strangulation. Strangulation occurs when a hernia twists upon itself and interferes with its blood supply, with ischaemia and necrosis developing within 6 hours. This can eventually result in perforation, which presents with a painful, rigid abdomen with pyrexia, tachycardia and vomiting.

August Richter, German surgeon (1742–1812).

16. EPONYMOUS FRACTURES (2)

E – Smith fracture
There are three eponymous fractures related to the distal radius. The most common is the Colles fracture – a fracture of the distal 2.5 cm of the radius with dorsal and radial displacement of the distal fragment (leading to the classic 'dinner fork' deformity). A distal fracture of the radius that extends to involve the joint (i.e. intra-articular) is known as a Barton fracture. A Smith fracture is an extra-articular fracture of the distal radius that results in the opposite deformity to the Colles fracture, i.e. volar (palmar) displacement of the distal fragment.

Abraham Colles, Irish surgeon and anatomist (1773–1843).
John Rhea Barton, American orthopaedic surgeon (1794–1871).
Robert William Smith, Irish surgeon (1807–1873).

17. X-RAY CHANGES IN OSTEOARTHRITIS

E – Subchondral sclerosis
Osteoarthritis is the most common form of arthritis, its incidence increasing with age. It occurs primarily in the weight-bearing joints. The primary problem in osteoarthritis is in the articular cartilage, with abnormal repair and remodelling.

The four characteristic X-ray changes in osteoarthritis are:

1. Narrowing of joint space (due to cartilage loss)
2. Osteophytes
3. Subchondral sclerosis (laying down of new bone)
4. Cyst formation

Rheumatoid arthritis is a chronic systemic condition which generally presents as a polyarthritis. It is characterized by inflammatory changes in the synovial membranes, which in turn destroys articular cartilage.

The four characteristic X-ray changes in rheumatoid arthritis are:

1. Narrowing of joint space
2. Soft tissue swelling
3. Juxta-articular erosions
4. Joint subluxation

18. PAEDIATRIC ORTHOPAEDICS (5)

D – Still's disease
Juvenile rheumatoid arthritis is an autoimmune arthritis of children (under the age of 16) characterized by joint inflammation for more than 6 weeks. Various forms of the condition exist.

Still's disease is a systemic form of juvenile arthritis characterized by intermittent high fevers and a transient generalized 'salmon-pink' rash.

Other features include arthralgia, myalgia, hepatosplenomegaly, lymph-adenopathy and pericarditis. The condition is most common in early childhood, although an adult form also exists. The systemic illness is self-limiting over a period of months, although chronic arthritis persists and may only present some time after the acute illness. Diagnosis is based on clinical findings and raised inflammatory markers. Rheumatoid factor and anti-nuclear antibodies (ANA) are usually negative.

Juvenile pauciarticular arthritis is the most common form of juvenile arthritis (60%) and usually affects young girls under the age of 8. It involves less than four joints and usually affects small and medium sized joints (knees, elbows, ankles and wrists). Joint involvement is usually asymmetrical and patients are usually ANA positive. There is a risk of developing anterior uveitis (30%). *Juvenile polyarticular arthritis* (30% of juvenile arthritis) affects five or more joints. It is similar to adult rheumatoid arthritis in that it is a symmetrical condition which affects both small and large joints. It is most common in teenage girls. Rheumatoid factor may be positive. Juvenile arthritis may be a relapsing and remitting condition or may take a chronic course. Treatment options include non-steroidal anti-inflammatories, disease modifying drugs (e.g. methotrexate), steroids and physiotherapy.

Sir George Frederic Still, English physician (1861–1941).

19. INVESTIGATING BREAST DISEASE (2)

E – Prolactin levels

Galactorrhoea in the absence of pregnancy or breast feeding must alert the clinician to suspect a prolactinoma. Prolactin is a hormone produced by the anterior pituitary gland which stimulates breast milk production and excretion in women. Its action is inhibited by dopamine. Prolactinomas are the most common benign tumours of the pituitary gland, and significant tumours occur at an incidence of around 1 in 7000. Presenting symptoms include those attributable to raised prolactin levels such as galactorrhoea, infertility and loss of libido in both sexes, together with amenorrhoea in women, and pressure symptoms from the tumour itself including headaches and visual disturbance (typically bitemporal hemianopia, caused by pressure on the optic chiasm). Prolactinomas are best visualized on MRI of the brain. Treatment of these tumours is dependent on their size, and includes dopamine agonists (bromocriptine), surgery and radiotherapy. Other causes of raised prolactin levels include hypothyroidism and some drugs (e.g. haloperidol).

20. COMPLICATIONS OF THYROIDECTOMY

B – Bedside opening of incision

Bleeding is a recognized complication following thyroid surgery (1%). Acute bleeding causing airway compromise is an emergency. If there is any suggestion of airway compromise in a post-operative patient, look for a haematoma. If present, it must be evacuated immediately, even before transfer to theatre. Further investigation is not needed. Other complications of thyroid surgery include damage to the recurrent laryngeal nerve causing vocal cord paralysis. If bilateral, this will result in respiratory distress following extubation. Unilateral paralysis presents later with hoarseness of the voice. The parathyroid glands, which produce parathyroid hormone that increases serum calcium, are situated posterior to the thyroid and may be damaged during surgery, causing hypocalcaemia. This results in circumoral paraesthesia and tetany, and may cause cardiac arrest. Another complication of surgery is the 'thyroid storm', in which manipulation of the thyroid gland leads to profound hyperthyroidism resulting in hypertension, tachycardia, hyperthermia and potentially fatal cardiac arrhythmias. If this occurs during surgery the first step is to discontinue the procedure. Beta blockers and propylthiouracil (a thyroperoxidase inhibitor) are used pre-operatively in thyrotoxic patients to prevent this occurrence. Hypothyroidism is expected at some stage following thyroid surgery. This must be diagnosed and treated early.

21. ANORECTAL DISEASE (4)

B – Condylomata acuminata
This patient has features of anal warts. Anal warts are caused by human papilloma virus (types 6 and 11) and are spread by anal intercourse. Warts are often asymptomatic but may present with itching, discharge or bleeding. On examination, pink and grey lesions may be seen around the anus and perineum. If these lesions are large and coalesce they are known as condylomata acuminata.

Condylomata lata are large, fleshy, white lesions that occur in the genital region with secondary syphilis.

Condylomata acuminata, from Latin *condylomata* = knuckles + *acuminatum* = pointed.

Lata, from Latin *lata* = broad.

22. SKIN LESIONS (5)

E – Pyogenic granuloma
A pyogenic granuloma is an acquired haemangioma (note, it is neither pyogenic nor a granuloma) which occurs most often on the head, trunk, hands and feet. It develops at a site of trauma (e.g. thorn prick) as a bright red nodule which bleeds easily and enlarges rapidly over 2–3 weeks. It affects those at the extremes of age but is most common in pregnant women. These lesions are benign and are managed by excision, although smaller lesions may resolve spontaneously.

Kaposi sarcoma is a malignant tumour of vascular endothelium that gives rise to plaques and nodules in the skin and mucous membranes that have a bruise-like appearance. It is associated with underlying human herpes virus 8 infection in people who are immunosuppressed (such as those with AIDS or patients taking immunosuppressants following organ transplantation). Before the advent of AIDS, Kaposi sarcoma was a rare sporadic tumour that occurred in male Italians and Ashkenazi Jews. Biopsy of the lesions is required to confirm diagnosis and symptomatic treatment is with radiotherapy.

A *ganglion* is a benign, tense, cystic swelling, often at the back of the wrist, that occurs due to degeneration of the fibrous tissue surrounding the joints. It is most common in young women. Ganglia are usually painless and asymptomatic although they may occasionally press on adjacent nerves (ulnar and median nerves). Asymptomatic ganglia do not require treatment, and many spontaneously resolve. Lasting cure is by excision (aspiration is simpler, but 50% will recur).

Moriz Kahn Kaposi, Hungarian dermatologist (1837–1902).

23. KNEE CONDITIONS (3)

E – Osgood–Schlatter disease

Osgood–Schlatter disease typically affects athletic adolescents and is caused by traction on the tibial tubercle at the point of insertion of the patellar tendon. It commonly presents as pain after activity or with a tender lump over the tibial tuberosity. It may be bilateral. X-rays are rarely indicated but may show fragmentation at the tibial tubercle. Treatment is with rest, analgesia and abstinence from sports until symptoms settle.

Chondromalacia patellae is also a cause of anterior knee pain in girls and is a result of softening of the articular part of the patella. Pain is typically worse on climbing the stairs and on standing from a seated position. *Dislocation of the patella* is acutely painful and caused by a twisting or direct injury usually with the knee in slight flexion. The patella can be felt at the lateral border of the knee. Dislocations may be recurrent. A *bipartite patella* is a congenital anomaly where the patella is made of two parts. It can be mistaken on X-ray for a fracture but it rarely causes pain. A *Baker cyst* is a swelling of the synovial sac of the knee joint which can be palpated in the popliteal fossa. It can rupture, resulting in acute knee pain and calf swelling.

Robert Bayley Osgood, American orthopaedic surgeon (1873–1956).
Carl Schlatter, Swiss physician (1864–1934).

24. GROIN LUMPS (5)

A – Epididymo-orchitis

Epididymo-orchitis (inflammation of the epididymis and testis) presents with a painful swelling of the epididymis with constitutional symptoms such as pyrexia and malaise. Patients may also exhibit a secondary hydrocele. Because epididymo-orchitis is usually a consequence of ascending infection (for example from a urinary tract infection or a sexually transmitted urethritis) there may also be a history of dysuria or urethral discharge. When someone presents with a painful, swollen testicle it is important to rule out testicular torsion – if there is doubt the patient should be referred for urgent surgical exploration. Treatment of epididymo-orchitis is with bed rest and a long course of antibiotics (e.g. 6 weeks of oral ciprofloxacin). If an abscess develops it requires drainage.

Mumps is caused by a paramyxovirus infection that is spread by saliva droplets and affects pre-adolescents. As well as constitutional symptoms, patients develop inflammation of the parotid glands (parotitis). Recognized complications of mumps include meningitis, pancreatitis and orchitis, from which there is a small risk of sterility. The incidence of mumps has been drastically reduced by routine administration of the MMR (measles, mumps, rubella) vaccine.

25. JAUNDICE (5)

E – Pancreatic carcinoma

Pancreatic carcinoma is the third most common malignancy of the gastrointestinal tract and is the fifth most common cause of cancer-related death. Its incidence increases with age, particularly after 50 years, and it is more common in men. Risk factors include smoking, diabetes mellitus and chronic pancreatitis. The most common site of malignancy is within the head of the pancreas (60%); around 20% arise in the body and 5% in the tail. The classic presentation of a carcinoma in the head of the pancreas is with painless progressive jaundice. Other symptoms include epigastric and back pain, pruritus, marked weight loss and thrombophlebitis migrans (recurrent clots in superficial veins). Patients may have noticed pale stools and dark urine. Jaundice occurs secondary to obstruction of the common bile duct, which results in a full, palpable gallbladder. Courvoisier's law states that 'if in the presence of jaundice the gallbladder is palpable then the cause is unlikely to be gallstones'. The prognosis of pancreatic cancer is very poor – a 5% survival at 5 years. The only chance of cure is by surgical resection of the tumour by Whipple procedure (removal of the pancreatic head, common bile duct, gallbladder, distal stomach and part of the duodenum), although no more than 20% of patients are suitable for this at presentation. Palliation of obstructive symptoms can be achieved with stent insertion through ERCP. Most patients die within 6 months of diagnosis.

26. URETHRAL INJURY

E – Retrograde urethrogram

This patient has presented with a urethral injury, as indicated by the presence of blood at the urethral meatus. Injuries to the urethra may be classified as anterior (penile and bulbar urethra) or posterior (membranous urethra). Causes of anterior urethral injuries include straddle injuries (as in this scenario), penile fractures and iatrogenic injury, e.g. by repeated attempts at catheterization. Posterior urethral injuries are more common and almost always associated with a pelvic fracture. Urethral injuries are more common in men (as they have a longer urethra). Presenting symptoms vary depending on the site of injury but include oedema and ecchymosis of the penis (in anterior blunt injuries), blood at the urethral meatus, a high-riding prostate (in pelvic fractures), scrotal haematoma, butterfly haematoma of the perineum (caused by extravasation of blood not contained within Buck's fascia) and haematuria. If a urethral injury is suspected then urethral catheterization is contraindicated (as this could damage the urethra further). Diagnosis is with a retrograde urethrogram, where a Foley catheter is gently placed into the urethra and injected with contrast. Extravasation of dye indicates urethral rupture. Following diagnosis, a suprapubic catheter is inserted and surgical repair can be performed (sometimes as a delayed procedure). Complications of urethral injury include stricture formation leading to difficulty in voiding, impotence and incontinence. In the multiply injured patient and in those with a pelvic fracture, a CT would be the most appropriate investigation in the first instance, with a retrograde urethrogram being performed once the patient is stable.

27. NECK LUMPS (5)

E – Thyroglossal cyst

A thyroglossal cyst is a congenital cystic remnant of the thyroglossal tract. It usually presents in the first decade as a smooth midline lump which moves up on tongue protrusion (note that thyroid lumps do not move up with protrusion of the tongue). Diagnosis is by ultrasound and treatment is by excision of the cyst and thyroglossal duct (Sistrunk operation).

Thyroglossal, from Greek *thyreoeides* = shield-shaped + *glossus* = tongue.

The thyroid was thought of as the shield-shaped gland.

Walter Sistrunk, American surgeon (1880–1933).

28. EAR DISEASE (2)

C – Cholesteatoma

A cholesteatoma is a pocket of stratified squamous epithelium within the middle ear which is expansive and locally destructive. It may be a congenital abnormality, but the majority arise as an acquired condition following trauma to the eardrum (e.g. perforation). The condition is more common in men. Presentation is usually with painless foul-smelling discharge (cholesteatomas are usually colonized with *Pseudomonas aeruginosa*) which is resistant to antibiotics, and conductive hearing loss. As the cholesteatoma progresses it can cause vertigo, facial nerve palsy or destruction of the mastoid, and give rise to cerebral abscesses. Otoscopy usually reveals a perforation associated with a central mass of debris within the middle ear. When investigating a patient with a suspected cholesteatoma it is important to get a CT to assess the extent of destruction. Treatment is by excision of the cholesteatoma and any destroyed tissue. Regular follow-up is required as cholesteatomas may recur.

Acute otitis media describes acute infection of the middle canal that most commonly occurs in young children following an upper respiratory tract infection. Common causes include *Streptococcus pneumoniae*, *Haemophilus influenzae* and *Moraxella catarrhalis*. Children present with ear pain and conductive deafness. On examination the tympanic membrane is red, dull and bulging, due to the build-up of pus. If the tympanic membrane perforates, the pain settles and purulent, blood-stained fluid will be seen discharging from the ear. Management of acute suppurative otitis media is with antibiotics (e.g. penicillin).

Glue ear is the name given to a chronic ear effusion. It is a relatively common finding in children. There is accumulation of non-suppurative fluid in the middle ear resulting in reversible conductive deafness. Affected children may suffer behavioural change and impaired cognitive development due to chronic deafness. On examination a dull tympanic membrane is seen in the absence of inflammation. Most cases of glue ear resolve spontaneously within 3 months. If symptoms persist beyond this, management is by grommet insertion.

Swimmer's ear is another term for otitis externa. Otitis externa is diffuse inflammation of the skin lining the external auditory meatus, often bacterial or fungal in origin. Features include outer ear irritation, scanty discharge and pain that is worse with jaw movement. It is most common in people with a narrow, tortuous ear canal and in patients who have traumatized the skin of the outer ear, e.g. by a towel or cotton buds. *Cerumen* (ear wax) is produced by the ceruminous glands of the outer meatus. Impaction of wax (e.g. by cotton buds) can result in conductive deafness. Management is by ear syringing.

Cerumen, from Latin *cera* = wax + *albumen* = white.

Cholesteatoma, from Greek *chafe* = bile + *steat* = fat; 'growth containing bile fats', as they often contain cholesterol.

29. TRAUMA

D – Immobilize the patient

The approach to any trauma case must follow the sequence: Airway (including C-spine immobilization), Breathing, Circulation, Disability and Exposure. Even though it is apparent that this patient is in shock and probably has a fracture of his left leg he must be immobilized to protect the cervical spine, and airway and breathing cleared before addressing the issue of blood loss and other injuries. Common sites of blood loss in trauma patients are the chest, abdomen, pelvis and long bone fractures. Temporary splinting, e.g. of the pelvis and long bone fractures, aids in preventing further blood loss while resuscitation is taking place.

30. ABDOMINAL PAIN (15)

A – Aspirin

This patient has presented with a perforated peptic ulcer. Spillage of stomach contents results in chemical peritonitis. The majority of peptic ulcers and perforations occur in the duodenum. Ulceration is the result of gastric acid and pepsin action on the mucosa. Predisposing factors include *Helicobacter pylori* infection, alcohol, smoking, regular use of NSAIDs (such as aspirin) and corticosteroid use. Gaviscon is used for the symptomatic relief of heartburn and omeprazole is a proton pump inhibitor which causes a long-lasting reduction in gastric acid production, being used in the treatment of ulcers.

31. CUTANEOUS MALIGNANCIES (3)

E – Squamous cell carcinoma

Squamous cell carcinoma (SCC) is a malignant tumour of keratinocytes that occurs in the over 50s in sun-damaged sites. Predisposing factors for their development include X-ray exposure, smoking, human papilloma virus and a genetic susceptibility. SCCs typically have raised everted edges with a central scab. Management is by surgical excision with lymph node dissection or radiotherapy if there is evidence of spread.

An *actinic keratosis* (solar keratosis) is a hyperkeratotic, yellow-brown crusty lesion that occurs on sun-damaged sites. These lesions are pre-malignant and may progress to SCC. For this reason actinic keratoses should be removed, e.g. by excision, shaving or cryotherapy.

A *keratoacanthoma* (or molluscum sebaceum) is a benign tumour of hair follicle cells. It occurs on sun-exposed sites (e.g. face and arms) and is more common in the elderly. Keratoacanthomas grow rapidly over 6–8 weeks and are characterized by a rolled edge with a central keratin plug which can fall out and leave a crater. Spontaneous resolution occurs but takes several months and leaves a deep scar. Keratoacanthomas are usually excised as there is a small risk of transformation to squamous cell carcinoma, and to avoid the deep scar. Squamous cell carcinomas are different to keratoacanthomas in that they grow slowly, there is no central core and they gradually ulcerate.

Bowen disease (or squamous cell carcinoma in situ) is a pre-malignant intraepidermal carcinoma with atypical keratinocytes. It typically occurs on the leg of older women. Bowen disease presents as large pink or brown flat lesions with a superficial crust that may look like eczema. Previous exposure to arsenic can predispose to the condition. A small percentage of these can progress to squamous cell carcinoma. Treatment is by excision. Erythroplasia of Queyrat is Bowen disease of the glans penis. It appears as a red, velvety lesion.

John Templeton Bowen, American dermatologist (1857–1941).

Louis Queyrat, French dermatologist (1872–1933).

Keratoacanthoma, from Greek *kerat* = horn + *akantha* = thorn; a thorn of horn.

32. MANAGING ENDOCRINE DISEASE (2)

B – Hydrocortisone and fludrocortisone

This woman presents with postural hypotension. She has vitiligo and some areas of increased skin pigmentation, which means she is likely to have Addison disease.

Addison disease is primary autoimmune-mediated adrenocortical failure. The adrenal cortex can be simplified as secreting three things: glucocorticoids, mineralocorticoids and adrenal androgens. These usually feed back to the anterior pituitary to reduce adreno-corticotrophic hormone (ACTH) secretion. Therefore if the adrenal cortex fails there are many consequences: reduced glucocorticoids (hypoglycaemia, weight loss), reduced mineralocorticoids (hyperkalaemia, hyponatraemia, hypotension), reduced adrenal androgens (decreased body hair and libido) and ACTH excess (increased pigmentation in sun-exposed areas, pressure areas, palmar creases, buccal mucosa and recent scars). The diagnosis of Addison disease is by the short Synacthen test. In this investigation, plasma cortisol levels are measured before, and half an hour after, administration of a single intramuscular dose of ACTH. Normally the ACTH will result in a rise in cortisol. If there is no rise in cortisol on the second reading, adrenal insufficiency is indicated. Management of Addison disease is with the replacement of glucocorticoids and mineralocorticoids (hydrocortisone and fludrocortisone respectively).

Thomas Addison, English physician (1795–1860).

33. PAEDIATRIC SURGERY (5)

E – Necrotizing enterocolitis

Necrotizing enterocolitis is a life-threatening infection most common in preterm children in the first few weeks of life. It is a non-specific infection of the bowel which may be secondary to hypoxia, fluid imbalance and septicaemia. There is an increased risk in children with patent ductus arteriosus. It has a lower incidence in breast-fed babies. Necrotizing enterocolitis can sometimes occur in outbreaks. Features include bile-stained vomiting, mucus and blood in the stools, and a distended erythematous abdomen.

Non-specific symptoms include lethargy, apnoea and shock. The diagnosis is largely clinical but may be aided by abdominal X-ray, which shows multiple dilated bowel loops. The treatment of necrotizing enterocolitis is supportive and includes total parenteral nutrition and broad spectrum intravenous antibiotics until the child improves. If there is any evidence of necrotic or perforated bowel, then laparotomy with bowel resection is indicated. Complications include malabsorption syndromes, stricture formation and the need for a stoma. There is an overall mortality of at least 10%.

34. UROLOGICAL CONDITIONS (2)

E – Vesica-ureteric reflux

Vesica-ureteric reflux is caused by an abnormal insertion of a ureter into the bladder resulting in the failure of the valves between the two. This results in the reflux of urine back up into the ureter on contraction of the bladder. Vesicaureteric reflux occurs in around 1 in 100 children and is more common in girls. If left untreated, it can result in hypertension and kidney failure. The degree of reflux varies from mild to severe (graded 1–5), where large amounts of urine are refluxing to the kidneys. Vesica-ureteric reflux can be bilateral. Treatment is with prophylactic antibiotics to prevent urinary tract infections and with early, aggressive treatment if infections do develop. If recurrent UTIs occur despite treatment, or reflux is present after the age of 5, then surgical re-implantation of the ureters is required.

A *pelvic kidney* results from incomplete migration of the kidneys and is rarely symptomatic. *Renal agenesis* is the failure of development of one or both kidneys. Most infants born with bilateral renal agenesis die within a few hours of birth, but unilateral agenesis rarely causes problems if the single kidney functions well. A *posterior urethral valve* is a cause of urinary tract obstruction in male children. *Hydronephrosis* describes distension of the renal pelvis and calyces.

35. FEMORAL NECK FRACTURES (2)

C – Hemiarthroplasty

The blood supply to the femoral head comprises the intramedullary vessels, the vessels in the retinaculum of the joint capsule and through the ligamentum teres (although at this age this may be obsolete). The choice of treatment largely depends upon the disruption to the blood supply caused by the fracture. Partial and undisplaced fractures through the femoral neck (Garden I and II fractures) may be fixed using a dynamic hip screw, as can intertrochanteric and subtrochanteric fractures. Minimally and completely displaced fractures (Garden III and IV) are likely to have severe disruption to the blood supply of the femoral head, leading to impaired healing and a risk of avascular necrosis; hence the head will need to be removed and replaced with a prosthesis (hemiarthroplasty). In fitter patients, a total hip replacement may be considered, but as this patient has dementia she is not a candidate. In younger patients (below the age of 60–65) much effort is made to preserve the femoral head, and open reduction and internal fixation is often attempted. In treating impacted neck of femur fractures, if not too painful, a watch and wait policy is sometimes adopted as healing may occur without intervention.

36. MANAGING BILIARY TRACT DISEASE (3)

B – Intravenous antibiotics

This patient has presented with acute cholecystitis, an acute inflammation of the gallbladder secondary to obstruction of the cystic duct. Ninety percent of cases are due to gallstones but in 10% no cause of obstruction is found (acute acalculous cholecystitis). Acalculous cholecystitis is most common at the extremes of age and is associated with major trauma, burns and surgery. Obstruction of the cystic duct results in chemical irritation (secondary to stasis of bile) and bacterial infection ensues. Symptoms of acute cholecystitis include upper abdominal pain, usually in the right upper quadrant, which may radiate to the back and shoulder tip. There is often associated vomiting. The presence of systemic upset, e.g. fever and elevation of inflammatory markers, helps to differentiate this from simple biliary colic. Murphy sign – pain on palpation below the right costal margin in the mid-clavicular line during inspiration – is a clinically useful sign (it can also be done with the ultrasound probe) but is present in only 40% of cases. Ultrasound investigation confirms the diagnosis. The treatment of acute cholecystitis includes intravenous fluids, intravenous antibiotics and analgesia. Symptoms usually resolve spontaneously within days without further intervention. Ongoing infection will result in an empyema of the gallbladder (a mass will develop as the gallbladder fills with pus) and this requires urgent drainage. Cholecystectomy is usually performed as an elective procedure 6 weeks after the resolution of symptoms (to reduce the risk of septicaemia) but may be performed as an emergency procedure if symptoms do not settle with conservative management.

37. MANAGING UROLOGICAL DISEASE (3)

E – Transurethral resection of prostate

Benign prostatic hyperplasia (BPH) is the most common benign neoplasia, characterized by the formation of nodules in the periurethral region of the prostate. At least half of all men have BPH by the age of 60 and its incidence increases with age. BPH results in bladder flow obstruction and symptoms include hesitancy, poor stream, and incomplete emptying of the bladder leading to frequency of micturition, nocturia and haematuria. BPH may also present with acute urinary retention. Long-standing obstruction can lead to bilateral hydronephrosis and renal failure. Specific investigations include urodynamic studies (assessing urinary flow rates) and the measurement of residual urinary volume. Treatment options in symptomatic patients include medical therapy and surgical intervention. Commonly used drugs include alpha blockers (e.g. tamsulosin), which reduce smooth muscle tone and decrease bladder outflow resistance, and finasteride (a 5-α reductase inhibitor) that inhibits the conversion of testosterone to the active dihydrotestosterone. Transurethral resection of the prostate (TURP) is indicated when medical treatment has failed; it is the most commonly performed operation in men and considered the 'gold standard' of surgical treatment in BPH. TURP involves shaving the inner portion of the prostate via a cystoscope. Specific complications of this procedure include impotence, retrograde ejaculation, incontinence and the need for a repeat procedure. If the prostate is very large, an open prostatectomy is preferred.

Radical prostatectomy, brachytherapy and external beam radiation are used in the treatment of prostate cancer. A bladder neck incision is made when urinary obstruction is secondary to hypertrophy of the muscles at the bladder neck.

Brachytherapy, from Greek *brachy* = short.

38. STATISTICS (3)

B – 50%
The positive predictive value (PPV) describes the probability that a condition can be confirmed given a positive test result.

PPV = (number of true positives/total number of positives) × 100

Thus,

$$PPV = (15/30) \times 100 = 50\%.$$

For other useful formulas, see the question 'Statistics (1)'.

39. MANAGEMENT OF VENOUS DISEASE (2)

D – Subcutaneous low molecular weight heparin
This man has developed a deep vein thrombosis, and may have secondary pulmonary embolism. Management can either be with intravenous heparin or subcutaneous low molecular weight heparins (LMWHs). Heparin requires a loading dose followed by a continuous infusion, and the dose of the drug is modified according to daily measurements of activated partial thromboplastin time (APTI). LMWHs are much easier to administer (by once-daily injection) and do not require monitoring. For this reason LMWH is the first-line treatment for deep vein thrombosis and

pulmonary embolism. Heparin is reserved for patients with severe, life-threatening thromboembolism. Treatment with LMWHs or heparin is continued until warfarin therapy has been commenced effectively.

40. MANAGEMENT OF AORTIC ANEURYSMS

D – Repeat an ultrasound scan in 3 months

The normal size of the abdominal aorta is 2 cm. A dilatation of the abdominal aorta above 3 cm is defined as an abdominal aortic aneurysm. Abdominal aortic aneurysms (AAA) are commoner in men, affecting 5% of those aged *over* 65 years. Other risk factors are smoking, hypertension, hypercholesterolaemia and a family history. The majority of AAAs (95%) are below the renal arteries (infrarenal) and 30% extend to involve the iliac arteries below. The risk of rupture of AAAs is directly proportional to the diameter. The risk of rupture of those AAAs with a diameter of less than 4 cm is low and so they can be followed up with annual ultrasound scans. AAAs with a diameter between 4.0 and 5.5 cm need to be followed up every 3 months. If the diameter is greater than 5.5 cm elective inter-vention is required unless the aneurysm is rapidly expanding (>1 cm/year), tender or symptomatic, in which case early repair is indicated. The mortality of elective repair of AAA is 5% as compared to a mortality of up to 50% in emergency cases, highlighting the importance of close monitor-ing and follow-up of even incidental AAAs.

41. MANAGING SKIN CONDITIONS (3)

B – Intravenous antibiotics and surgical debridement

This patient has necrotizing fasciitis, a rare but life-threatening soft tissue infection which spreads rapidly across fascial planes leading to oedema, vascular occlusion and tissue necrosis. The most common organisms responsible are the group A beta haemolytic streptococci, although other bacteria (*Staphylococcus aureus, E. coli*) may be isolated and some cases are polymicrobial in origin. Necrotizing fasciitis can occur after surgery or minor trauma, or the cause may be unknown. Risk factors include immunosuppression and diabetes mellitus. These cases present acutely with severe pain, systemic upset and progressive tissue destruction. Intravenous antibiotics, together with debridement of necrotic tissue, are required as soon as possible to prevent septicaemia, amputation and death. Mortality is around 25%. Polymicrobial necrotizing fasciitis of the scrotum, penis or perianal area is known as Fournier's gangrene.

42. COLORECTAL OPERATIONS (2)

C – Hartmann procedure

This man has developed peritonitis following perforation of a diverticu-lum. He will require an appropriate resection with a delayed anastomosis, known as Hartmann procedure. Hartmann procedure involves resection of the rectosigmoid colon with closure of the rectal stump and formation of a colostomy. This operation avoids the potential complications of forming an anastomosis under sub-optimal emergency conditions, when there is a greater risk of post-operative anastomosis breakdown. The colostomy can then be reversed at a later date.

For descriptions of the other colorectal operations listed, see the question 'Colorectal operations (1)'.

Henri Albert Hartmann, French surgeon (1860–1952).

43. TUMOUR STAGING

B – Dukes B

The Dukes system of grading colorectal cancer was originally divided into stages A, B and C. The modified Dukes system added a 'D stage', which describes the presence of distant metastases.

Dukes A	→	confined to the bowel wall
Dukes B	→	invade through the bowel wall but there is no lymph node involvement
Dukes C	→	invade the bowel wall and involve lymph nodes
	→	C1 = apical node not involved
	→	C2 = apical node involved
Dukes D	→	distal metastases present

Other examples of staging systems include:

Ann Arbor	→	lymphoma
Breslow	→	malignant melanoma
Gleason	→	prostate cancer

Cuthbert Dukes, English pathologist (1890–1977).

44. HAND DISORDERS (3)

C – Infective tenosynovitis

Infective tenosynovitis describes the infection of the tendon sheath, usually caused by direct penetrating trauma. The cardinal features of tendon sheath infections are summarized by Kanavel signs: (1) tenderness over the flexor sheath; (2) pain on passive extension; (3) flexed posture of the digit; and (4) fusiform swelling of the digit. The tendon sheaths of the thumb and little finger communicate with the radial and ulna bursa respectively, so infection of these sheaths will spread to the respective bursa. In at least 50% of people there is communication between the ulna and radial bursa, providing a further route of spread for infection (horseshoe tenosynovitis). Treatment may initially be with a period of intravenous antibiotics but drainage must not be delayed if there is no improvement.

Fascial space infections may affect any of the four potential spaces/compartments within the hand: the dorsal subaponeurotic space, the subfascial web space, the thenar space and the mid-palmar space. Infections within the former two compartments present with pain and swelling on the dorsum of the hand. Thenar space infections present with pain and swelling over the thenar eminence (lateral half of the palm) and the thumb will be flexed and abducted. Mid palmar infections present with swelling and tenderness in the centre of the palm, and a loss in the concavity of the palm will be apparent. Treatment is initially with antibiotics and elevation, but if there is poor response then incision and drainage is required.

Paronychia is an infection which occurs between the lateral nail fold and the pulp of the finger. It presents with localized pain and swelling. Infection may track to form a subungual abscess (infection between the nail plate and nail bed). Paronychia can result following minor injury while cutting nails, prolonged submersion in water and covering up of the digits for excessive periods of time. Treatment is with either antibiotics or antifungals as indicated; sometimes drainage is required. A *felon* is an infection within the closed space of the pulp of the finger. As compartments within the distal phalanx are small, increased pressure within these spaces caused by ongoing infection can lead to necrosis of the skin and finger pulp. Infection is usually the result of minor cuts. Treatment is with antibiotics and surgical decompression of any abscess. A *whitlow* is an infection of the skin and fibro-fatty pulp of the finger caused by the herpes simplex virus. In the initial stages, the tip of the finger is red and exquisitely painful, and this precedes the formation of vesicles. Treatment is with antivirals.

Paronychia, from Greek *para* = next to + *onyx* = nail.

Allan Buckner Kanavel, American surgeon (1874–1938).

45. GASTROINTESTINAL POLYPS (2)

B – Hamartomatous polyp

The association of circumoral freckling with multiple duodenal polyps is known as Peutz-Jeghers syndrome, a rare autosomal dominant condition. These polyps are benign hamartomas (a growth that is made up of the same tissues from which it arises).

Johannes Laurentius Peutz, Dutch physician (1886–1957).

Harold Joseph Jeghers, American physician (1904–1990).

46. BACK PAIN (3)

D – Spinal stenosis

Chronic back pain is the leading cause for time off work and causes significant disability. Causes of pain include trauma, degeneration, infection and malignancy. Spinal stenosis is the term given to narrowing of the spinal canal, most commonly caused by osteoarthritis. It may be thought of as a spinal claudication, as symptoms are caused by a lack of blood supply to the cauda equina in the restricted spinal canal. Symptoms are typically relieved by sitting or bending forwards, as these actions widen the spinal canal and help improve the circulation. Diagnosis is best made on MRI.

Spondylosis is the most common cause of back pain and is attributable to osteoarthritic degenerative changes leading to loss of height of the vertebrae and displacement of the posterior facet joints. The lumbar spine is usually affected in the L5/S1 and the L4/L5 regions. Pain is characteristically aching in nature and worse in the mornings and following activity. *Spondylolisthesis* is the spontaneous displacement of a vertebral body upon the one below. It commonly occurs at the L5/S1 region then at the L4/L5 region. Displacement is usually anterior. Back pain is usually worse while standing. A 'step' deformity may be felt on palpating down the spine. *Ankylosing spondylitis* is a seronegative inflammatory degenerative condition which largely affects the spine and sacroiliac joints. It is most commonly found in Caucasian males and associated with HLA-B27. Progressive fusion of the spine causes a 'bamboo spine' appearance on X-ray. *Spinal tumours* in adults are mostly metastatic in origin (e.g. from breast, lung and prostate). Pain is usually unremitting and associated with systemic features such as weight loss and night sweats.

47. URINARY TRACT INFECTION

B – *Escherichia coli*

Cystitis usually presents with dysuria, frequency of urine, suprapubic discomfort and fever. Cystitis is much more common in women due to their shorter urethra. *Escherichia coli,* usually found in the bowel, is the most common pathogen responsible for uncomplicated cystitis in the UK (75%). Cystitis can be confirmed by the presence of leucocytes, nitrites and blood in the urine. A mid stream urine (MSU) sample should be sent to microbiology for microscopy, culture and sensitivity. A positive culture is when more than 105 of a single organism are grown per millilitre of urine. The growth of mixed bacterial species usually indicates contamination of the sample. Antibiotic treatment should be guided by local patterns of bacterial resistance and MSU sensitivity results. Uncomplicated cystitis is usually treated with a 3–5-day course of trimethoprim. Other antibiotics that are used to treat cystitis include amoxicillin, ciprofloxacin, cefradine and nitrofurantoin. Patients who are susceptible to recurrent urinary tract infection can be prescribed prophylactic antibiotics (e.g. 100 mg of trimethoprim once nightly). Patients should be advised to drink lots of fluids and avoid dehydration. UTIs in men and children require further investigation to rule out an underlying structural problem.

48. MANAGING COMMON FRACTURES (3)

A – Administer further analgesia and call senior orthopaedic doctor on call

This patient appears to be developing compartment syndrome, an orthopaedic emergency commonly seen with long bone fractures, either secondary to the fracture itself or caused by a tight plaster cast. The senior orthopaedic doctor on call must see the patient. Compartment syndrome is caused by increased pressure in the osteofascial compartment leading to swelling, venous engorgement and later to arterial compromise and ischaemia. If left untreated, necrosis can develop within 12 hours leading to muscle death, contractures and irreversible nerve injury. Initially the only finding is increased pain that is out of proportion to the injury, with increase in pain on passive extension of the muscle compartments and some sensory deficit. Pallor, pulselessness and paralysis are late features of compartment syndrome and diagnosis must not be delayed until these features are present. Urgent decompression of the limb is required, and if compartment pressures are greater than 40 mmHg urgent fasciotomy is indicated.

49. UPPER LIMB NERVE LESIONS (4)

B – Axillary nerve

This boy presents with an anterior shoulder dislocation. The axillary nerve wraps around the surgical neck of the humerus and is damaged in 5–10% of anterior dislocations. It can also be affected in fractures of the humeral neck. The axillary nerve supplies the deltoid muscle and gives rise to the lateral cutaneous nerve of the arm (which supplies sensation to the upper, outer arm). Axillary nerve lesions result in anaesthesia in the upper, outer arm (the 'regimental badge patch' area) and paralysis of the deltoid muscle, resulting in limited arm abduction. While the arm cannot be abducted, if it is passively lifted above 90°, the arm can be held in abduction due to the action of supraspinatus.

The spinal root of the accessory nerve (cranial nerve XI) supplies the trapezius and sternocleidomastoid muscles. It can be damaged during dissections of the neck. Features of accessory nerve palsy include weakness of shoulder shrugging and the inability to turn the head against a force applied by the examiner.

The long thoracic nerve of Bell supplies serratus anterior, a muscle which helps stabilize the scapula. This nerve can be damaged during breast and axillary surgery, radiotherapy and axillary trauma. Lesions of the long thoracic nerve result in winging of the scapula, where the scapula becomes prominent on pushing the arms against resistance.

Sir Charles Bell, Scottish anatomist and surgeon (1774–1842).

50. ULCERS (4)

B – Cushing ulcer

A Cushing ulcer is the development of acute peptic ulceration in the setting of raised intracranial pressure, e.g. after intracranial bleed or traumatic brain injury. These ulcers most commonly develop within the antrum of the stomach, although the first part of the duodenum may also be affected. It is thought that ulceration is secondary to stimulation of the vagus nerve within the brain, leading to increased gastric acid secretion. The development of Cushing ulcers is known as the Rokitansky-Cushing Syndrome.

A *Curling ulcer* is an acute ulcer of the duodenum that occurs a few days following severe burns. The reduced plasma volume following burns injury results in necrosis of the gastric mucosa, with ensuing ulceration and perforation. *Decubitus ulcer* is another name for a pressure sore. These develop secondary to continued pressure on the skin from lack of mobility, leading to skin necrosis and breakdown. They commonly occur over bony prominences, e.g. ischial tuberosities, sacrum and malleoli. *Dendritic ulcers* are painful corneal ulcers caused by herpes simplex type 1. They are visible with fluorescein staining and have a characteristic 'branched' appearance, giving them their name. A *Martorell ulcer* is an ischaemic ulcer of the leg above the ankle that occurs secondary to hypertension.

Decubitus, from Latin *decumbere* = to lie down, related to *cubitum* = elbow (lie on your elbow).

Dendritic, from Greek *dendron* = tree (as in branched).

Thomas Blizard Curling, British surgeon (1811–1888).

Harvey Cushing, American neurosurgeon (1869–1939).

Fernando Martorell Otzet, Spanish cardiologist (1906–1984).

Karl von Rokitansky, Austrian pathologist (1804–1878).

Index